# HYDRATE TO ELEVATE

Electrolyzed Reduced Hexagonal
Water – The Key to Good Health

## DR. DEBI PRASAD ACHARJYA

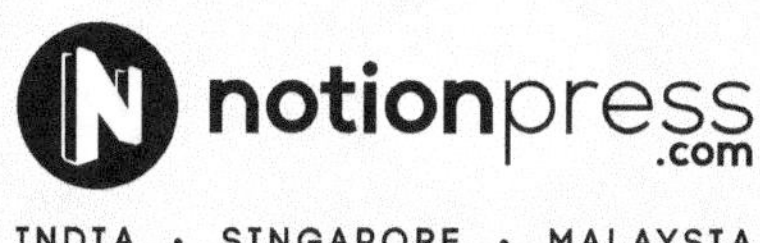

ISBN  979-8-88749-932-1

# MEDICAL DISCLAIMERS

- The information in this book does not replace your personal physician(s). It is an attempt simply to educate on certain things that your doctor may not have time to do. You must always look to your primary physician as your basic and final advisor for medical care and emergencies. Always work with a qualified healthcare professional before making any changes to your lifestyle, diet, prescription drug use, and exercise activities.

- The chapters and the articles are general in nature, and you are a specific and unique individual with unique needs and circumstances. One person's opinion does not reflect the opinion of all. This information should not be used to diagnose, treat, or cure any disease. One should consult their own medical professional(s) for more information.

- The information on the benefits of "Electrolyzed, Reduced, Hexagonally Structured and Alkalized Water" may not be supported by conventional medicine. However, they are well documented and supported by many physicians and health care professionals globally.

- Individuals suffering from any disease or illness should consult with a qualified physician or health care provider prior to beginning any of the treatments, therapies, supplements, or protocols mentioned. Utilization of these, or of any of the data and information in this work, implies acceptance of these disclaimers.

- Every known health challenge has its core and something to do with hydration. This is a critical piece of health puzzle. While going through this book, please keep in mind that you will not be discovering a cure to anything, except maybe dehydration. A superior form of water that renders to the body everything that it needs to heal, given enough time.

- There is nothing strange or unusual about this information and their consequences except that many of the treatment protocols is not recognized by the FDA and the Insurance Companies and thus is not commonly used or understood.

- It must be clearly understood that the information shared is not intended to diagnose or claim to prevent, treat, mitigate, or cure any health conditions. In presenting this information, no attempt is being made to provide diagnosis, care, treatment, or rehabilitation of individuals, or apply medical, mental health or human development principles, to provide diagnosing, treating, operating, or prescribing for any human disease, pain, injury, deformity, or physical condition.

- Many quotations are included as reference of what others wrote, said, or personally experienced to assist the reader in evaluating the potential of Hydrogen Water Therapy.

- Any references, company names, organization names or logos may not be endorsements of any specific product, service, company, or their opinion.

- It might well be possible that some of the website links mentioned in this book may not be available subsequently.

- The writer himself does not practice medicine nor has a practicing license and does not diagnose, treat, or advise sick or diseased patients. Kindly relate accordingly.

- Any liability, loss or risk that may be incurred therefore, directly or indirectly, from the use or application of the contents of this book is specifically disowned.

# CONTENTS

# ACKNOWLEDGEMENTS & DEDICATIONS

Let me acknowledge that the life-changing information shared within the pages of this book is not my original work. In fact, I am just another ordinary man who happened to find my way through and learn a series of extraordinary knowledge and wisdom revealed by some of the greatest masters in the field of Health and Wellbeing.

This book might serve as a tool for the Professionals associated with the Wellness Industry (and the ultimate end users) for enriching their knowledge on Hydrogen Water Therapy and the benefits of the Water Ionizers for a pro-active living.

The information, suggestions and references provided in this book is based on the resources freely available on the electronic and print media. The articles are designed just to provide competent and reliable educational information regarding the topics covered. However, it is presented with the understanding that the writer is not a physician by profession and not engaged in rendering professional advice nor it is intended to discredit the medical fraternity.

It must be clearly understood that the information shared is solely intended to present alternate views and not to diagnose or claim to prevent, treat, mitigate, or cure health condition.

This book is the direct result of OPW: Other People's Wisdom; My gratitude to those who have personally shined their light of wisdom before me, and to the greats (some no longer with us) from whom I have benefited through their magnificent writings: You have inspired me, motivated me, and given me the information I need to make this the most effective, fulfilling life possible, both for me and for those whose lives I am fortunate to touch.

In essence, I am only a chosen instrument on a mission to propagate some of these incredible "Wellness Secrets" to special people like you and possibly make a difference in your life. Whatever I have learned, I am thrilled to share it with you.

Over the years, I have learned that an unconditional willingness to acknowledge the source is one of the true signs of growth and leadership. For this reason, I consider it is my duty to acknowledge these remarkably special people in my life with utmost honor and humility.

I acknowledge Dr. Jerry Tennant, Dr. David Jockers, and Dr. Joseph Mercola among others. I have extensively quoted their findings in this book. A special mention must be made of "Molecular Hydrogen Institute (MHI)." MHI does not represent, endorse, or recommend any specific hydrogen products/companies. The contents of this book have NOT been evaluated by MHI. This book is the outcome of my learning with MHI when I was introduced to this fascinating world of Hydrogen.

In fact, everything that I have been able to accomplish in my fulfilling life has been a direct result of what others have challenged me to do, taught me to do, supported me through, coached and mentored me all the time and at times even innovatively jeered at me to accomplish. I would like to acknowledge them too for helping me bringing out the best in me.

Importantly, I consider any piece of my work, may it be a book, a seminar, a piece of art, a business, a relationship, a career or even my very own family, as a "body of work". It is simply an embodiment of many great minds, intense experiences, incredible teachings, sensible mentoring, priceless sacrifices, and never-ending learning on the part of many who have touched my life in one way or the other.

# WATER AND THE HEALTH PUZZLE

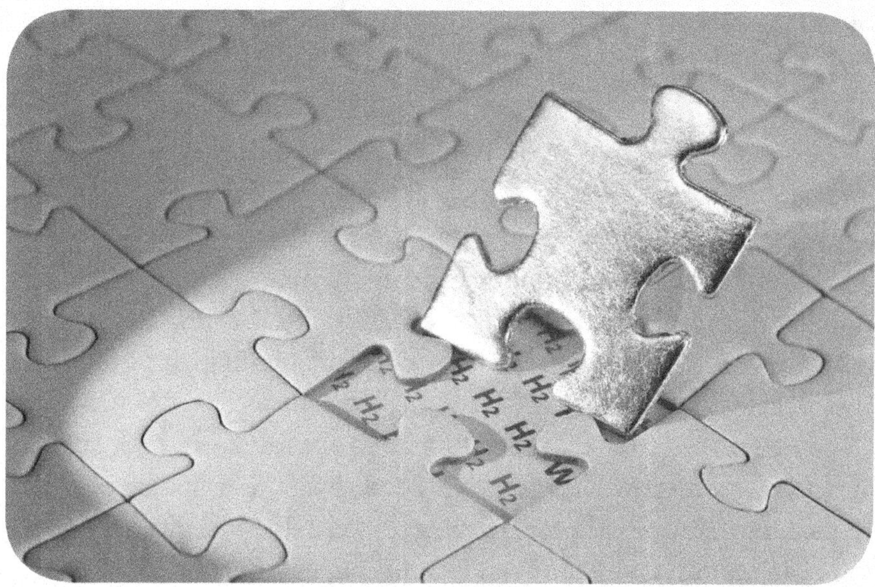

The water we consume was and continues to be 70% of our health puzzle. Without it, the other 30% that we work so hard on, will not be effective.

Changing my water helped me overcome persistent health challenges and it literally changed my life!

I have carefully compiled detailed information about a special type of water and its healing properties. These, I am sure, will inspire you and help your clients / patients immensely.

And if you are a healer, you need more time to recover than most. We give so much of ourselves that we often forget to take care of our own selves. It is earnestly hoped that the stress and frustration of being in practice and the healthcare arena would be diminished.

There will be lots of valuable information that will be shared about water and its healing properties. When you first start looking into the real research, it can feel a bit overwhelming. It may be quite possible that even after undergoing extensive education on healing, attending 100's (even 1000's) hour sessions, you might not have heard about Electrolyzed Reduced Water (ERW). This might make you feel unsettled.

Water is an extremely complicated subject to research. There are several reasons for this. First, there is a wide variety of water forms such as: Distilled, Reverse osmosis, Filtered, Alkaline, Ionized, Alkaline Ionized etc.

However, the hardest one to find is the one with an enormous amount of clinical research. It is called **ELECTROLYZED REDUCED WATER**. You can also research its components like the Molecular Hydrogen, Oxygen, Hydroxide, and the Aquaporin.

You then need to find legitimate sources of material and not fall into the marketing realms. The internet is flooded with information on water all claiming cure and all of them having personal financial interests. These will certainly not serve your quest for authentic information.

The sites that I use predominantly are the **PubMed** and **NIH**, but other medical journals also have the most recent research. Still better, you can visit **google.scholar** which provides a simple way to broadly search for scholarly literature.

Another aspect to become aware of is that these sites contain all the research from the beginning of time. In the 70's, distilled water was conceptually amazing, later research determined the inherent dangers negating the prior research.

You can pick any subject or topic: Cancer, Diabetes, Inflammation, Brain, Multiple Sclerosis, Parkinson's, Inflammation, etc. I have outlined few of the most helpful research links in this book.

There are so many more ways that we can help our potential clients. Not only is there good clinical research out there supporting

Electrolyzed Reduced Water, but there are vast quantities that have been studied for decades!

It is like discovering a buried treasure, a lost secret to the fountain of youth that had been hidden long ago. The truth is... we are all 70% or more, water.

Every known condition has at its core, something to do with hydration. Electrolyzed Reduced Water is a critical piece of the health puzzle, and with it chances of the body getting back to balance are much greater. This statement is validated by research, details of which are available all throughout the book.

Keeping those things in mind, we have not discovered a cure to anything, except maybe dehydration. A superior form of water that renders to the body everything that it needs to heal, given enough time.

> *"You're not sick, you're Thirsty.*
> *Don't treat Thirst with Medication."*
>
> *- Dr. F. Batmanghelidj, MD*

We must realize that healing is almost never one thing. But rather, it is a finely tuned combination of several things, if not a great many things.

The information that is being shared is not designed to diagnose, treat, or to be used in lieu of qualified medical attention. These little pearls of wisdom come from actual application of the different types of electrolyzed reduced water by me personally for more than 6 years of continuous use and innumerable personal testimonies from patients under supervision of his/her personal physician, based with a specific outcome that is expected and monitored.

The reality of the power of Electrolyzed Reduced Water is... JUST DRINK THE WATER!

The Electrolyzed Reduced Water, with other waters, from the "Water Ionizing Generator" which I have been using since the last 6 years has been approved as a Medical Device by the Japanese Ministry of Labor and Welfare. Additionally, these Ionizers have been given the Seal of Approval by The Japanese Association of Preventive Medicine for Adult Lifestyle Diseases. This association comprises of more than 6,500 Japanese Physicians and Surgeons. These are also GOLD SEAL Certified by the Water Quality Association (WQA), USA. Being an Original Equipment Manufacturer, they are associated right from the research, and finally till the distribution of their products to the end users globally. With a 48-year history, they initially provided ionized, alkalized water to hospitals in Japan since 1974 for 20 years before being introduced as a domestic unit.

No health claims are made through this book. Please also note that I am not a physician. This is a modest attempt to highlight little information which can benefit the readers. Collectively through awareness, education, and knowledge we can be effective in our health and longevity. Being a conscious individual, you are advised to make your own decisions. All of us are entitled to health and prosperity.

Drinking Electrolyzed Reduced Water will help you feel the difference right away – inside out. I can assist you to own this amazing piece of technology which renders ordinary tap water into Electrolyzed Reduced Water which brings the body back to balance.

Thanks, and Regards.
**Dr. Debi Prasad Acharjya**
(Wellness Consultant & Hydration Specialist)
D. Hon., Diploma in Cellular Nutrition Therapy (DCNT), B.Sc. (Gold),
Hydrogen Advisor (Molecular Hydrogen Institute)

# ELECTROLYZED REDUCED WATER FOR GENERAL WELLNESS

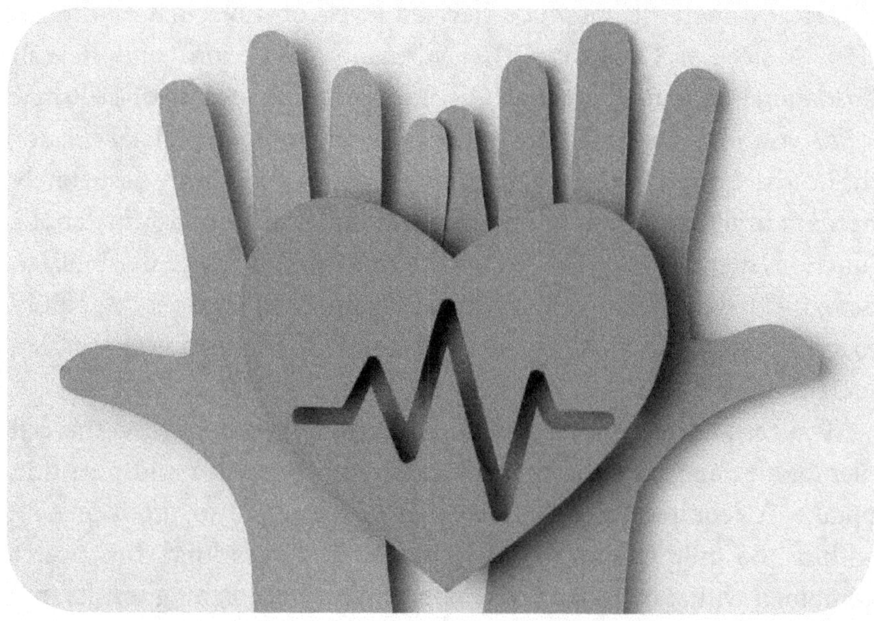

Electrolyzed Reduced Water (ERW) is water that has been electrically altered (charged) verses chemically altered water (adding chemicals/minerals). The electrolysis process that the water undergoes, produces "stable" water ionization at a high enough level that it breaks the bonds between the $H_2O$. The shift in alkalinity is an indicator that the process has occurred; the pH itself is irrelevant for the most part because it is not chemically induced.

As you know, you can change the pH of water simply by adding calcium, magnesium, potassium, or even regular baking soda, etc. ERW is not the same thing as alkaline water.

**All ERW is alkaline but not all alkaline water is ERW.**

Electrolyzed Reduced Water is exactly that, water that has been broken apart, restructured, and made more bio-available to the human body using electricity.

When the water ($H_2O$) goes through the electrolysis machine, it is electrically altered to produce elevated levels of Molecular Hydrogen ($H_2$), Molecular Oxygen ($O_2$), Hydroxide ($HO^-$) ions and has an Oxidation Reduction Potential (ORP) approaching (negative) – 800 mV.

As you may know, the lower the ORP, the more beneficial it is for the human body. It is these above four things that our body desperately needs to function normally. If you wish to increase the body's metabolic function, increase its ability to uptake nutrition, increase its ability to detoxify the cell from cellular metabolism that increases the ability to exchange $O_2$ and $CO_2$, you must check if these four things are increasing or not.

The reason our body requires Hydrogen ($H_2$) is to feed the cell membranes and increase their permeability to oxygen and nutrition uptake. It requires increased levels of oxygen ($O_2$) to produce ATP within the mitochondria. Early research shows that this water combined with a hyperbaric chamber renders astonishing results that have required the charts for oxygen uptake be rewritten. The body also requires hydroxide anions ($HO^-$, antioxidants) which are used to flush the toxins of cellular metabolism out of the body. At last, it requires a high electric potential (ORP) which is the electrical charge as well as the energy that the body uses to make everything work.

I would like to briefly discuss a couple key areas where a significant level of research is available. There is a health crisis sweeping the entire globe regarding cancer, diabetes, and neurological disorders. If we can find **any** option to significantly improve the odds with these conditions, it will be a great step forward. As we just discussed the four main components of the water, $H_2$, $O_2$, $HO^-$, and ORP, each of these aspects individually play a key role in the above stated conditions.

Many people misquote Dr. Otto Warburg who originally won the Nobel Peace prize for his clinical research on cellular respiration, the mitochondria, and cancer. What he found was that if a cell were deprived of oxygen by 35% for over a 48-hour period, the mitochondria would shut down or stall the Krebs cycle and the cell would start to burn sugars, reverting to glycolysis. As you are aware, a healthy cell produces 34-36 ATPs during a normal Krebs cycle. However, glycolysis drops that efficiency down to 4 units of ATP. The phenomenon that leads to a cell becoming cancerous has been shown by the Warburg research. To validate this, it was said that increasing the level of available Oxygen at the Mitochondria and increasing the electron potential can help reverse this shut down of the mitochondria.

Cancer is such an aggressive disease process that is extremely challenging to manage. It requires **multiple avenues of treatment**. All these aspects are further complicated by the individual being treated, history, health habits, compliance, etc. It is in these areas that we can increase our ability to help by rebuilding the body from inside and increasing our success rates.

Neurologically, hydration plays a key role and has a dramatic effect on the brain and nervous system for both mental and emotional function. Neurologists agree that of all conditions involving the brain, 60+% of the issue directly involve dehydration.

The elevated levels of dehydration of the brain and the nervous system relates to their intense need for molecular hydrogen and oxygen. Because ERW has some of the highest levels of dissolved oxygen and hydrogen, it is no surprise that there is an immense level of clinical research pertaining to the health benefits. It ranges from something as simple as proper brain hydration stabilizing the levels of cellular metabolism to rebuilding the myelin sheaths that help protect the nerves themselves.

Diabetes is another common condition that responds extremely well to the application of ERW. One of the predominant features is the fact that ERW can rapidly detoxify the intra-cellular matrix. This works at reducing the insulin resistance due to the build-up of metabolic waste within the cell itself. We have seen some amazing results pertaining to sugar spikes, glucose levels, and drops in insulin usage.

A diabetic client can suffer from ulcerations and there is a phenomenal solution to this. The Electrolyzed Hypochlorous Acid has been used as a sterilizing and healing agent for diabetic ulcers, neuropathic ulcers, gangrene, necrotizing fasciitis, etc. for decades. It is a FDA approved sterilant for durable medical and dental devices, and potent sterilant for nearly everything from MRSA to E.Coli. The ability to easily and affordably all but eliminate cross-contamination cannot be underestimated. The ramification for the clinical application of Electrolyzed reduced Hypochlorous Acid to the wound care and sterilization may well revolutionize the whole industry.

There is a level of clinical research out there in NIH and PubMed that directly ties Electrolyzed Reduced Water to the treatment of cancer, diabetes, a wide range of neurological conditions, and other disease processes.

While I have mentioned a few research links (at the end of this chapter) for you to review, I would encourage you to do more research for yourself. A simple PubMed and/or NIH search for Electrolyzed Reduced Water is usually enough for most of us. But the pertinent question remains – "Why is it that I am not aware about this before?" Personally, I was also overwhelmed at the level and quantity of the research out there.

Further "Molecular Hydrogen ($H_2$) Research" articles are available for the individual disease conditions. You can do your research on Electrolyzed Reduced Water (ERW) at **https://scholar.google.com/**

Hope that this answers some of your basic questions and spurs you on to asking more questions and doing more research. I am not a physician and do not treat patients. This is just a synopsis or a summary of my learning about ERW. Kindly relate accordingly. It is to be clearly understood that whatever discussions and the health benefits for any health challenges listed here, the Electrolyzed Reduced Water should not be taken as a standalone line of treatment. **No medical claims are made through this book.**

## Articles for Review:

ERW Inhibitory Effect on Tumor angiogenesis
https://www.jstage.jst.go.jp/article/bpb/31/1/31_1_19/_pdf

ERW Suppressor2 stage cell formation
https://pubmed.ncbi.nlm.nih.gov/19003049/

ERW delays mammary tumor growth
https://www.ncbi.nlm.nih.gov/pmc/articles/PMC6196883/

ERW and Oxidative damage
https://www.ncbi.nlm.nih.gov/pmc/articles/PMC4212634/

The Neuro-protective effects of ERW
https://www.ncbi.nlm.nih.gov/pmc/articles/PMC3285010/

ERW protects neural cells from oxidative damage
https://www.ncbi.nlm.nih.gov/pmc/articles/PMC4212634/

Suppressive Effects ERW on Type1 Diabetes
https://pubmed.ncbi.nlm.nih.gov/21063772/

Preservative effects of ERW of pancreatic beta-cells
https://pubmed.ncbi.nlm.nih.gov/17268057/

Hypochlorous Acid: an ideal wound care agent with powerful microbicidal, antibiofilm, and wound healing potency
https://pubmed.ncbi.nlm.nih.gov/25785777/

Potent Wound Care Agent
https://www.ncbi.nlm.nih.gov/pmc/articles/PMC1853323/

Future GOLD standard for wound care
https://pubmed.ncbi.nlm.nih.gov/31904191/

Cardiovascular Effect of electrolyzed high-pH alkaline water on blood viscosity in adults
https://www.ncbi.nlm.nih.gov/pmc/articles/PMC5126823/

Daily ingestion of alkaline electrolyzed water containing hydrogen influences human health, including gastrointestinal symptoms
https://www.ncbi.nlm.nih.gov/pmc/articles/PMC6352572/

Effects of Alkaline-Reduced Drinking Water on Irritable Bowel Syndrome with Diarrhea: A Randomized Double-Blind, Placebo-Controlled Pilot Study
https://www.ncbi.nlm.nih.gov/pmc/articles/PMC5925025/

# THE LIFE-CHANGING PROPERTIES OF HYDROGEN WATER

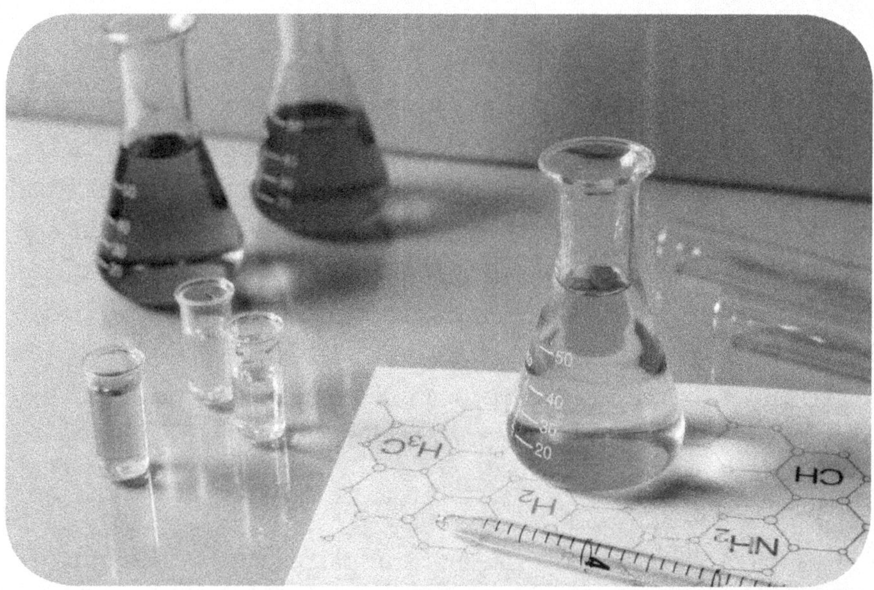

In 2015, Dr. Shigeo Ohta, Department of Biochemistry and Cell Biology, wrote about Molecular Hydrogen as a Novel Antioxidant with advantages for Medical Applications in which he stated with conviction: "Hydrogen rapidly diffuses into tissues and cells… We propose Hydrogen for prevention and therapeutic applications… for many diseases."

Everyone's body has various degrees of toxicity. Therefore, the effects of Hydrogen water on our body will be different for individuals. It will all depend on the diets of our past and the present, our hydration habits, and our exercise regimen. Then we need see the levels of stress in our lives and the loads of medicines we have taken thus far and as a result how toxic we have become. Regardless of all these, Hydrogen water can be life changing or even lifesaving for all of us who drink it every day.

The very first thing that Hydrogen water does when we begin drinking is it cleanses our digestive tract. This is one such process which has the potential to significantly improve our health for the better. It is simply not possible to assimilate the nutrients if the digestive tract is not at its prime. During the process of digestion, the enzymes attack the chemicals on the food and break them down. This process continues till they can pass through the linings of our small intestine and finally get absorbed into our blood. Once there, nutrients are carried to our liver and other body parts to be processed, stored, and distributed. Little to none of this happens if your digestive tract is not clean of waste and debris.

When we start drinking Hydrogen water, the first thing it does that it starts cleansing our digestive tract leading to a better health.

## Detoxifying

Our intestines can become museums of partially digested, putrefied foods, drugs and other toxins that never found their way out of our body. If our small (upper) intestine is not cleaned and their wall lining is not exposed, nutrients cannot get into your blood stream for our body to use. Ionized Hydrogen Water is a superb cleanser for digestive tract because the tiny Nano-size bubbles (dissolved Molecular Hydrogen gas) can be infused into the water by an Ionizer. Additionally, Hydrogen gently cleans as our GI tract while it also hydrates out tract's lining, so that the nutrients can pass into our blood with greater ease.

When this occurs, assimilation of nutrients into our body returns and initial stages of cellular rejuvenation starts to begin. When first drinking Ionized Hydrogen Water, people comment how often they go to the washroom. This is good because Hydrogen water is fully cleansing our digestive tract, organs, joints, tissues, joints, skin, and bones. It will gradually subside after your body is used to drinking Hydrogen water every-day.

## Alkalizing

Drinking Hydrogen Alkaline water reduces our body's all-round acidic levels as it balances is our body's overall pH, which is best measured through our urine or saliva. However, raising our overall body pH will take some time. Acid waste did not accumulate throughout our body overnight and it will not be flushed out overnight. Many years of accumulated acid waste in our joints, around our organs, in our brains and throughout our body takes months and even years to completely expunge. Of course, how quickly we cleanse our body of acid based also depends on our diet.

## Oxygenating

All bodily functions depend on oxygen for cellular respiration. Our cells need oxygen for two functions: (a) to produce Adenosine Triphosphate (ATP), the energy-carrying molecule found in the cells of all living things. The chemical energy obtained from the breakdown of food molecules is captured by ATP which is then released to fuel other cellular processes; (b) to eliminate toxins and waste through oxidation.

Our lungs consume about 5-6 milligrams of oxygen per minute, and we breathe out about 12-20 times per minute. Over the course of a day, that adds up to 17,000 to 30,000 breaths per day - or more (at rest)! Through our lungs, oxygen enters a capillary network and is bonded to hemoglobin (a protein molecule in red blood cells). Our red blood cells transport oxygen. The red blood cells contain oxygen-binding hemoglobin molecules and in case of poor blood circulation, there is a reduced delivery of oxygen. When viewed under a microscope, conventional water moves or blood red blood cells slowly. In contrast, Hydrogen water moves our red blood cells rapidly throughout our body. So, drinking Ionized Hydrogen water can increase our blood oxygen delivery, energy levels and elimination of toxins.

## Antioxidant

There is a constant battle inside our body between elements that are oxidative and antioxidant. Hydrogen water is rich in antioxidants and bathes our body in the lightest liquid for human consumption. Hydrogen promotes rejuvenation of each bodily system at a sub-cellular level; the antioxidant enzymes – Glutathione, Superoxide Dismutase, Catalase etc. gets activated.

Antioxidants are associated with anti-aging. Hydrogen gas has antioxidant properties. We can slow down and/or reverse aging by drinking Ionized Hydrogen water. We will not become 20 years old again, if we are 40 years old. Rather, we can possess the body we had when we were there in our twenties at the cellular level. The cells that make up our body can be as active, productive, functional, and communicative as those we had in our prime. Thus, we have reversed our biological clock, not our chronological clock. Like and older home that needs remodeling, or body can gradually be "remodeled" to feel like its younger self… month-by-month… year-by-year as we daily drink plenty of Hydrogen water.

## Hydrating

After we drink ionized Hydrogen water for a while, we become more sensitive to when we are dehydrated. Our body sends signals and makes us aware that it needs water, within an hour of not drinking any water. By keeping your body constantly hydrated, we accomplish many things that are necessary to achieve great health. When we are hydrated, our blood is never too thin or too thick due to lack of water or salt. Most of us do not retain salt nor have high blood pressure when we drink plenty of healthy Hydrogen water. Our organs function optimally because they are not starved for water, especially your kidneys.

Like any muscle, regular use of Hydrogen water will strengthen our kidneys. There is a common misconception that drinking too much water leads to overburdening of our kidneys. If you have weak kidneys from dehydration or living on nutrient-poor diet, start by drinking freshly ionized Hydrogen Alkaline water with the 7.5 pH to 8.5 pH range. Provide your body with a full array of nutrients from real foods and drink plenty of Hydrogen Alkaline water. The weak kidneys can become powerful, flexing muscles again. This is true of any muscle or organ in our body.

# MOLECULAR HYDROGEN FOR OPTIMUM HEALTH – THE SECRET MYSTERY OF AGING

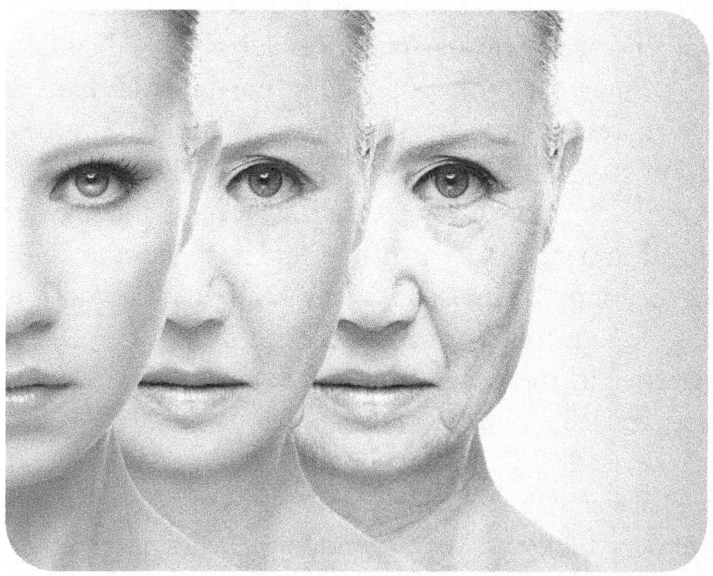

We are programmed to get old and look old, but it does not have to be that way. We see people who are 65 look like 45. Similarly, people who are 65 may look like 85. Age and Longevity are relative.

We inherit genes from our parents which plays an important role in our physical and mental attributes. We just cannot deny this fact. But we can make efforts to improve the quality of our lives as without this, life will not be exiting. We need to believe that we can make a significant difference and eventually act.

The prime thing is to know and understand what we are putting inside our bodies. We are starving and hydrating ourselves to death by consuming nutritionally junk food and vacant water, thereby getting fatter and sicker than before.

What is happening is that we are consuming tasty foods that are loaded with calories and produce energy... they do not have any nutritional value. We are starving ourselves to death by consuming these beautifully packaged, ready-to-eat dead foods.

Empty foods as described above do not produce nutrition. Instead, they build and accumulate as poison in our body and wastes in our blood. Accumulation of these toxins in our body leads to diseases (common expression of accumulated toxins) and can be the beginning of our death.

We very often cause disease ourselves. Sickness and low quality of life go hand in hand. There is neither life nor vitality in antibiotics, flu shots or immunization. Life, beauty, and youth are in the blood and good blood is made of good food and good water. Diseases are not manifested by themselves and cannot be cured by itself with the lifestyle we created for ourselves.

We make our living on white breads, cookies, pastries, cakes, and pretty package commercial foods sold at supermarkets. Then include all the tens of thousands of preparations including most so-called "health foods" and "healthy cereals." Add to these the foods that have been chemically treated and made look beautiful in appearance... fried, impaired, and impoverished foods... pasteurized and/or dead foods. Can we expect good blood, vigorous health, and stamina if we live on these foods?

One of the main causes of aging and disease can be found in the derangement of normal processes of cell metabolism and cell regeneration. The accumulation of toxins (from acidic foods, waters, beverages, and other sources) and metabolic waste products interferes with nourishment of our cells and slows down health cell regeneration and healthy new cell building.

Due to the nutritional deficiencies, our normal metabolic process gets derailed leading to sluggish digestion and elimination, sedentary life, overeating, acidosis etc. The process of cell nourishment, rebuilding, and replacement slows down and our body starts aging. Its resistance to disease will diminish and various ills will start to appear. So, an early key to anti-aging is shifting our overall body pH to being slightly alkaline.

Choosing the right food, living waters and hydration fluids to put in our bodies is the key to long life, strength, beauty, and youthfulness. It all sounds so simple, but it is not. Food is not necessarily healthy food and water is not necessarily healthy water.

So let us now begin our journey towards the Wonderful World of Hydrogen!

We are extremely fortunate to be alive during a global movement towards "Hydrogen Water Therapy" and enjoy its abundant health benefits. Hydrogen was present at the dawn of time, and it is the father of all known elements in our Universe. In our galaxy, hydrogen is the most abundant gas. Earth could not sustain life without it because almost 70% of our planet's surface is covered in water (Two Hydrogen Atoms + One Oxygen Atom = $H_2O$). Our human body is a "bag of $H_2O$." Science, for centuries, has overlooked the possible health benefits of the "$H_2$" in $H_2O$.

We have few millions of hydrogen atoms in the glass of water we drink. But the question arises is how those 2 Hydrogen atoms attached with the 1 Oxygen atom of $H_2O$ be separated from the water molecules? Secondly, how can we get these millions of liberated singles Hydrogen atoms pair with each other and forming a very safe and emerging medical gas, permeate into a glass of water?

Humans have survived for 90 days without food. But we can live only 72 hours without water before going into a semi-comatose state.

However, drinking water that is saturated with inorganic minerals such as magnesium carbonate, calcium carbonate and other elements our bodies cannot use, may lead to a variety of unhealthy conditions and diseases.

These inorganic minerals, toxic chemicals, fluoride, and other contaminants can pollute, clog up add even turn our tissues to stone, causing pain, illness and even premature death. Hydrogen water, the healing water, removes inorganic mineral deposits and toxins from your joints, and may remove cholesterol and fat. It creates a pH balance in our body. This book unlocks the mysteries of Hydrogen water which can help us relieve chronic suffering. Using the miracle of "Hydrogen Water Therapy" can help us live healthier, happier, and longer life.

Get introduced to what may be the greatest discovery in medical science and health care since 1953.

*"Hydrogen has Therapeutic Potential in 170 Disease Models, and in essentially Every Organ of the Human Body."*

*- Tyler LeBaron,*
*Molecular Hydrogen Institute / International Society of Hydrogen Medicine, and Biology.*

# ACIDITY – FATHER OF ALL DISEASES (AND ALKALINITY CONQUERS DEATH)

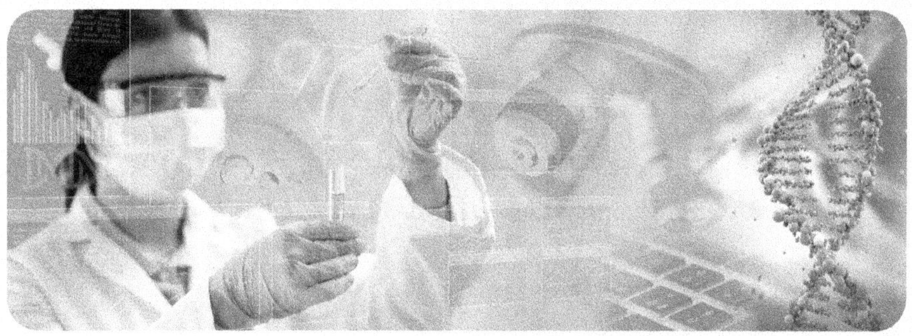

Accumulation of acidity in our blood, cells, tissues, organs, and body fluids can be a principal factor and/or cause of disease and death. Leading researchers suggest there is no natural death. They believe that deaths due to "natural causes" are the ending stages of progressive acidic saturation leading to toxemia in our bloodstream.

Most of all foods we eat are acid forming and it is just not possible to mention about them all. Almost all processed foods are acid forming. Most bottled products, including bottled waters, are acid forming. The modern cooking oils, bottled and attractively packed jams, jellies, syrups, all sugar items (sweets), cereals are acid forming. Foods which are fried, baked and even cooked, nearly all of them are acid forming.

Almost all drugs, pills, patent medicines, drinks, tonics, wines, liquors, coffee, tea, chocolate, cocoa, and all manufactured foods are acid forming. Nearly all canned fruits are acid forming. All nuts are acid forming except almonds. Most peppers and pickles are acid.

Acid forms as the product of our own metabolism (catabolism). Catabolism is our set of metabolic pathways that breaks down molecules into smaller units that are oxidized to release energy or used in other anabolic reactions. The products of combustion or oxidation in our body are acid forming. The dying leukocytes, the dying tissues, the excreta in the bowels, the mucus, phlegm, dying bacteria and their toxins are all acid forming. Even brain activity, thinking, worry, temper and all sorts of unfavorable emotions usually result in acidity.

> *"There is no natural death. All deaths from so-called natural causes are merely end point of a progressive acid saturation."*
>
> *- Dr. George W. Crile*

When our bodies are alkaline, it is more difficult to get sick. It is easier to get sick when our bodies are acidic. Human alkalinity and longevity go together. Human acidity can often lead to inflammation, pain, suffering, disease, surgeries, and an early funeral. However, an alkaline diet with alkaline hydration results in better health, anti-aging, and beauty.

None of us can escape wrong choices. If we live on acid-forming foods meal after meal, our body must eventually pay the price. As acid forming foods accumulate, blood toxemia can gradually develop. When blood toxemia teaches a tipping point, death will often knock on our door. Therefore, acidity is a foundation of many diseases, trouble, misery, pain, and tears.

Acid in or around the nerves can result in neuralgia, sciatica, nervousness, nerve pain, headache, earache, or various nerve elements. Acid brain matter can result in inflammation of the brain, insanity, crime, violent passion, melancholia, and hundreds of mental disease symptoms. An acidic brain cannot function normally.

Acid can cause arthritis, urinary ailments, heart valve issues and kidney problems. Acidity in or around the prostate gland can cause enlargement of the prostate, swelling and hardening, resulting in prostate cancer, or at the very least, urinary difficulties. An acidic uterus can lead to female complications of the menstrual cycle, inflammation, uterine tumors, and other ailments of the generative organs.

An acidic liver may result in constipation, piles, hepatitis, gallstones, and cirrhosis of the liver. Excessive acidity in our stomach can cause gastritis and heartburn. Acidity can cause gas generation and gas pressure upon our heart, diaphragm, spine, and other organs.

But there is hope! We are beginning to realize that in the conventional medical and pharmaceutical establishments of the corporate level is dependent on us for its profits. There is always a conflict of interest in this system.

It is not our intention to disrespect any doctors or healthcare professionals. We hold in high-regard and have very deep respect for the most conventional doctors, surgeons, nurses, clinicians, and other licensed health-care providers. This global community of dedicated professionals has spent many years saving lives by means of their study, hard work and long hours and hospitals and the field.

Different diets have different effects on our health. But an acidic-dominant diet always has a harmful effect on our body. One chemical body type is subject to one kind of acidity and other chemical body type is subject to another kind of acidity and gas formation.

There are many kinds of acid responses depending on the biochemistry of our unique and individual bodies. An important first step is to learn what an acidic food is along with an acidic water or beverage and what is an alkaline food and alkaline water or beverage. This is because human alkalinity and longevity go hand in hand.

## Alkalinity Conquers Death

As we grow older it is ever more important to know the properties of food and beverages including waters so that we make selections that are alkaline. As per Dr. Bernard Jenson we must consume a diet of 80% alkaline foods and 20% acidic foods to achieve "green inside" goal. As we live longer, there is danger of excess acid formation and gas generation. Poor elimination, low vitality, tissue acidity and autointoxication all come with age because of our ignorance and of acidic and alkaline foods or beverages.

When we are alkalized or balanced, there is virtually no excess acidity, no gas, no autotoxins, no poisons and no accumulation of blood toxemia. Oxygen is abundantly supplied. Our brain and nerves are well nourished and our red blood cells flow vigorously to all parts of our body. Then we can regain biological youth and enjoy a great quality of life. We can help speed up this process by drinking freshly ionized hydrogen alkaline water in our daily routine.

If we aim to change our diet and fluid intake before we are 90% dead, we can start reversing the aging process which is often a disease of poor diet and dehydration. Frequently, aging can also be called a disease of progressive acid saturation. Because we are "programmed" to grow old, and die does not mean that it is natural. Changing our diet and drinking ionized alkaline hydrogen water can help slow this deterioration and, in many cases, stop this deterioration.

Acid forming foods, which should be temporarily limited during the alkalizing period, are principally meat, fish, poultry, eggs, cheese, fat, white bread, starchy foods, cakes, pastry, candy, white sugar, and confections. It is best to avoid these or taken in quantities that do exceed our body's requirement needs.

# pH AND THE INTELLIGENCE OF OUR SUB-CELLULAR HEALTH

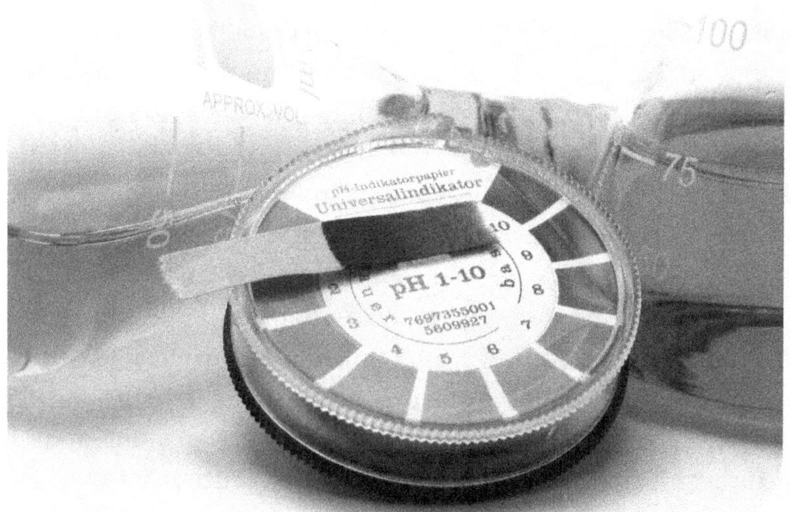


The abbreviation pH stands for power of Hydrogen. The total pH scale ranges from one to fourteen, with seven considered neutral. Any reading above 7 is therefore alkaline and any reading below 7 is considered as acidic.

If the body is at a slightly alkaline state, it will function at its best. Deviations in our blood above or below a pH range of 7.35 to 7.45 can signal serious symptoms of diseases. In physiology, if someone has a blood pH of 7.1, they are said to have acidosis even though, technically, 7.1 is slightly alkaline. If blood pH drops below 7.0, our body will not survive very long. In fact, when the levels of our cell tissue move away from the healthy state into the acidic state (especially below 7.0), the acidic wastes normally back up, as in a clogged sewage system.

The pH of blood, tissues and bodily fluids affects the state of our cellular health. We will always feel elevated feelings of wellbeing and vibrant health when there is a balance in our pH levels. Every metabolic and organ/system function depends on our delicately balanced pH, including all regulatory mechanisms such as digestion, metabolism, respiration, hormone release, neurotransmitter release and immunity.

It is important to understand that pH of blood is critical to our lives and survival. The pH of the blood has a very small degree of tolerance for variation. Our body does everything in its power to keep it within a slightly alkaline "healthy" range. This range, between pH 7.35 to pH 7.45, is maintained by pulling alkaline minerals such as calcium out of our bones and other body stores, if necessary.

If our body is overwhelmed by excess acids from poor diet and hydration habits, or over-exposure to chemical and environmental toxins… built-in compensating mechanisms go into effect to neutralize and excrete acidic toxins from our blood, cells, lymph, and tissue fluids. There are multiple internal buffering systems our body uses to neutralize acids and balance pH. If this neutralizing mechanism (buffers) becomes overwhelmed and cannot function adequately, the excess acid will severely compromise our cellular function, eventually causing a complete metabolic and system breakdown. This might ultimately lead to serious health problems, even cancer.

> *"The battle between life and death and humanity's struggle with sickness is over pH"*
>
> *- Dr. Gary Tunsky*

We live and die at the sub-cellular level. All our body's 37.2 trillion cells need to be slightly alkaline and must maintain this alkalinity to function and remain healthy and alive. However, their cellular activity creates acids which is the source of energy for the functioning of the cells. As each alkaline cell performs the task of respiration, they excrete metabolic wastes, and these end products of our cellular metabolism are acidic in nature.

These wastes are used for energy and function and are not to be allowed to build up. Most people and clinical practitioners believe that our immune system is our body's first and foremost line of defense. But some medical researchers are learning that it is not. Of course, our immune system is vitally important. However, it is more like a very sophisticated clean-up service. Instead, we can adapt to the Hydrogen Water Therapy along with the pH balance maintained at a slightly alkaline level as a major treatment option against disease and sickness.

What is killing us? The reason might well be "acidosis." Fungus, mold, bacteria, and viruses thrives in an acidic environment if the body lacking in oxygen (anaerobic). Research supports this fact.

Calcium makes up 1.5 % of our body weight. It is literally the human glue that holds to our bodies together. The biggest problem scientists have found is that over time our body becomes depleted of calcium.

There are chemicals (calcium) which aids a buffer for our blood. This buffer maintains alkaline level (or lack of acidity) in our blood. Without it we would die. If the pH level in blood moves even slightly towards acidic, we can get extremely sick. But to supply calcium for buffering, we must have enough calcium absorbed from our diet, waters and beverages or a body will simply extract needed calcium from our bodies and teeth.

Our human body is highly intelligent. It has a strategy to protect our vital organs from acidity which irritates, inflames, and scars them. Fat cells can be used to store some toxins and acids from metabolic processes that are trapped in our body by lack of water. These toxins can be seen by the dark black or brown fat that comes out during liposuction. So, some (not all) toxins and acids are stored in fat cells.

When acid contacts an organ, it can eat holes in our tissue. This may cause some of the cells to mutate. Oxygen levels drop in this acidic environment and calcium is depleted. The human body now acts to make fat to defend and protect us from the toxicity on account of acidic self. To do this, the fat cells may mop up the acid and take it away from our organs. Temporarily, our fat may save our vital organs from damage. But that fat will cause so many other health problems.

Osteoporosis is very confusing for many people. They think that it can be eliminated by increasing their consumption of milk and dairy products. But in countries where consumption of dairy products is low… the instance of osteoporosis is rare. Osteoporosis is often related to acidosis. As our body becomes more acidic, to protect against the event of heart attack, stroke, illness or even cancer, our body steals calcium from our bones, teeth, and tissue. When bone mass becomes depleted, that is osteoporosis. In simple terms what it means that by utilizing our very own calcium (which was stolen earlier), the body raises the pH level towards alkalinity to protect itself.

One warning sign of being too acidic is an appearance of calcium deposits. Did you know there has never been a science-proven association between calcium deposits in the body and nutritional calcium? In fact, just the opposite is found in the results of testing calcium deposits in our bodies. Calcium deposits come from the structural calcium of the bones and teeth and from dietary calcium.

When our body is overwhelmed by acidosis-toxicity, mechanisms are triggered to neutralize build-up of poisonous acids to maintain a slightly alkaline pH. Alkaline solutions (pH over 7.0) absorb oxygen, while acids (pH under 7.0) expel oxygen. Excess acid gives our body fluids less ability to access and absorb existing oxygen. This is a spiral downward into disease. More access to existing oxygen in our body via Hydrogen water gives our body fluids the ability to absorb more oxygen. This is an upward spiral towards health.

# HOMEOSTASIS VIA THE "HYDROGEN WATER THERAPY"

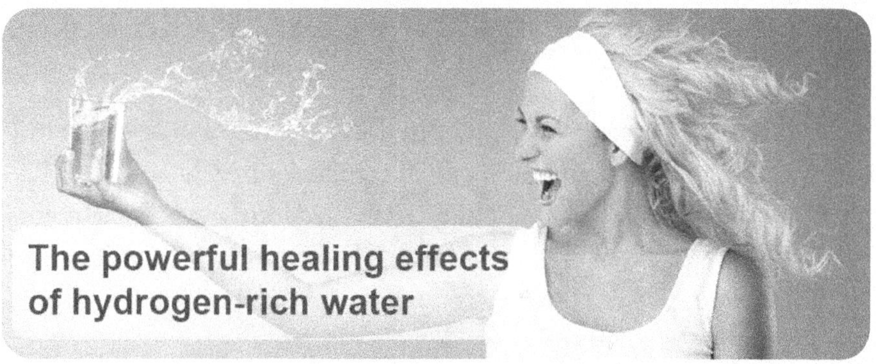



Hydrogen is an emerging medical gas with unlimited potential to restore homeostasis to virtually every organ of our body. In simple terms it is the condition of seeking for maintaining dynamic equilibrium within a cell or our entire body. It requires constant adjustments as conditions change inside and outside of us via complex feedback loops.

When our overall body achieves homeostasis, we feel stable, healthy, vibrant, and sometimes even younger because each of our body systems contributes to homeostasis of other systems.

Here are four main examples of homeostasis inside our bodies:

- Regulates amounts of water and minerals in our body (osmoregulation); this happens primarily in the kidneys.
- Removes metabolic waste (excretion); this is done by excretory organs such as our kidneys and lungs.
- Regulates blood glucose level; this is mainly done via our liver with insulin and glucagon secreted by our pancreas.
- Regulates body temperature; this is mainly done by our skin.

## The First Key for Optimal Health – Homeostasis

Did you notice how water participates in all four examples of homeostasis? Almost each one of us assumes that mostly blood is flowing through our 60,000-mile circulatory system. But you will be surprised to learn that only about 12% of fluids moving through your "blood stream" are blood! The other 88% is water (+/-) for average adult.

- Average percentage of water in the total body mass of a healthy adult body is about 60% (+/– for gender or age).
- Fluid distribution in our body is divided into two compartments – first the intercellular, which has about twenty-eight liters and second, the extracellular, which has about 14 liters (for a total of about 42 liters).
- Total blood volume (plasma, white blood cells and platelets) is about 5 liters.

So, 5 liters of blood divided by 42 liters of water fluid is equal to 11.9%. Is it not interesting? I am sure you were not aware of this fact. We are truly "skin bags" of water. Essentially every bodily system and each organ need water to achieve its own homeostasis.

Here are just a few examples that are not precise, since they can vary from person to person along with each person's ever-changing internal conditions:

Eyes: 95%, Liver: 70-75%; Bones: 31%; Lungs: 83%; Brain & Heart: 73%; Hair 10-13%; Muscles & Kidneys; 79%; Skin: 64%; Teeth: 8-10%.

"Hydrogen Water Therapy" offers the simplest solution for a vibrant health by combining healthy purified water with hydrogen, the smallest and the lightest molecule in our Universe.

Here are a few of our bodily functions that require healthy water:

- For our survival and digestion, it converts the foods to its components.
- To manufacture hormones and neurotransmitters needed by our brains.
- Forms saliva.
- To Keep our mucosal membranes moist.
- Regulates body temperature (sweating and respiration).
- The body cells are allowed to grow, reproduce, and survive.
- For our brain and spinal cord, it acts as a shock absorber.
- Flushes out body waste, mainly in urine.
- Helps lubricate our joints.
- Oxygen gets delivered all over the body.

The "Hydrogen Water Therapy" has three sought-after properties:

- Studies demonstrate its high safety profile.
- Therapeutic potential in hundreds of diseases.
- Offers a simple universal approach to personal home health care... because everybody already drinks water.

## Benefits of Molecular Hydrogen Therapy

No matter how young, strong, or healthy we may think we are… an appearance that our body is healthy does not guarantee that we are disease-free. Disease can get a foothold in our body without our awareness.

Below are just some of the many conditions and diseases people suffer or can be "suddenly" diagnosed with:

High blood pressure; High cholesterol; Acid reflux; Irregular bowels; Tumors; Arthritis and osteoporosis; Kidney stones, Migraines, Dementia; Parkinson's disease; Kidney disease; Influenza and pneumonia; Diabetes; Respiratory disease; Heart disease; Cancer... to name the major few.

**All of us need "Molecular Hydrogen Therapy" primarily for prevention**. Why wait for a sudden diagnosis we can have a revolutionary personal home health care system that proactively protects and prevent diseases from, in many cases, not even starting? And at the same time, this healthcare system can also be reactively used for treatment.

## Absorption – The Final Key to Hydrogen Water Therapy Success

Homeostasis is the first key to optimum health with water and hydrogen. Now let us complete our circle of success by learning how vital absorption is.

We can eat and drink the healthiest food and liquid on earth, but if their nutritional and hydration properties are not fully completely absorbed by our body, we can still get sick, experience a serious health problem or even a disease develop inside us.

Complete absorption is when our body can absorb via our intestine nearly 100% of healthy foods and liquids. Our digestive system is a marvel of engineering. It works as under:

An average person consumes about two liters of water daily through drinking water or via food or other beverages. Also, the volume of gastrointestinal secretions (including salivary, gastric, pancreatic, bile juice and intestinal) amounts to around eight liters. Therefore, a total of about ten liters of fluids (water based) gets passed through our intestines each day.

Liquids without chewing take the same route as food. We swallow liquids; they pass through our esophagus into our stomach where they wait for upper intestine to open via our pyloric valve. It is a thin circular muscle surrounding the pyloric opening in the first segment of our upper GI tract. Our pyloric valve appears to be pH sensitive and react in a variety of ways under a variety of stomach conditions.

Remember that at least ten liters of water-based fluids pass through daily which equals 3650 liters every year. Our upper intestine is about twenty feet and has an inner surface area of nearly 250 square meters, which is the size of a tennis court. This large surface is for quick and efficient absorption of water and other fluids. Little wonder our upper intestine absorb about 90% of our water.

Having understood the above, please go through the following information very carefully:

Like all cell membranes, our intestinal cells have a lipid bilayer that is about 5 to 10 nanometers thick. It is this barrier that marks our cell boundaries. The cell membranes of nearly all living organisms and many viruses are made of lipid bilayer, as are the membranes surrounding the cell nucleus and other sub-cellular structures. These bilayers are impermeable to most water-soluble molecules. Bilayers are particularly impermeable to ions and ionic bonds, which allow cells to regulate salt concentrations and pH by transporting ions across their membrane using proteins called ion pumps.

Most polar molecules (electro-negativity between two atoms is about 0.5 to 2.0) have low solubility in the core of a lipid bi-layer... and... have low permeability (absorption) characteristics across the bi-layer.

Hydrogen is the smallest molecule in our Universe and the purest covalent bonding non-polar molecule (electro-negativity between 2 hydrogen atoms is near 0.0). Therefore, Hydrogen can safely and easily pass through the lipid bilayer along with healthy water and minerals. We now have water that can be fully absorbed at the cellular, sub-cellular, nano and/or epigenetic levels. Research supports the above statements.

One published article shows hydrogen gas increases gastric emptying, which is faster absorption, via increased ghrelin secretion.

Please refer the clinical study effects of bicarbonate-alkaline mineral water on gastric functions given below*.

Hope you have now understood the significance of this "Hydrogen Water Therapy?"

It helps delivery and complete absorption of hydrogen infused water, safely to our bodies, which gives the therapeutic and disease fighting results.

Are you excited about this medical-science discovery? Every month, more global doctors, scientists, researchers, and other health professionals embrace "Hydrogen Water Therapy" as a great discovery and integrate it into their medical practice and personal home health care program.

Hopefully, you might have understood why this Hydrogen Water Therapy can be considered as the greatest discovery in medical science and health care since 1953.

In review, let us summarize its primary benefits:

- Restores homeostasis to our body systems and organs.
- Regulates and removes at sub-cellular levels.
- Demonstrates highest safety profile.
- Prevents or treats hundreds of diseases.
- Prevents universal approach to personal home health care.
- Shows no reported noxious side effects.
- Provides a proactive therapy for disease prevention.
- Offers fastest and deepest absorption rates.
- Supported by an ever growing global medical and science community.

*Hydrogen → Homeostasis → Absorption → Optimum Health*

---

* [https://www.ncbi.nlm.nih.gov/pubmed/16772353](https://www.ncbi.nlm.nih.gov/pubmed/16772353) (2006)

# THE ULTIMATE LIFETIME HEALTH INSURANCE POLICY

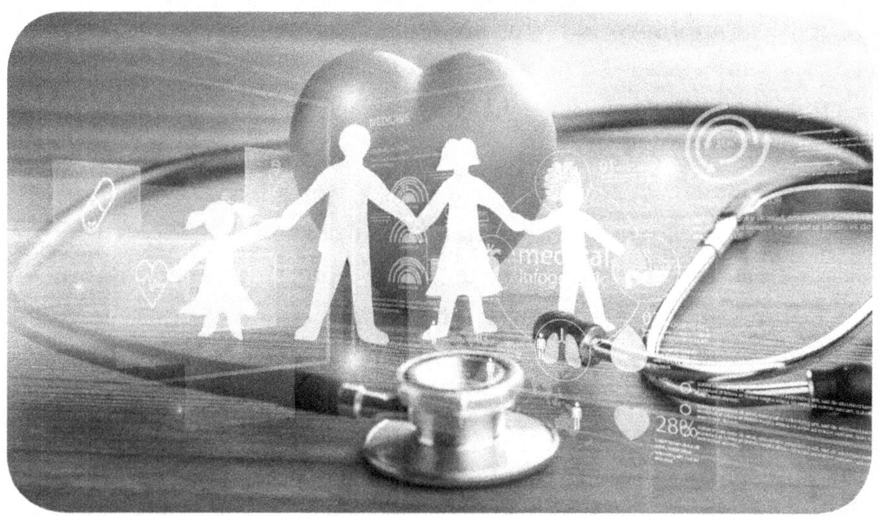

## "You are healthy until you are not healthy."

This means, we can be healthy one day (for many years or even decades) and that can suddenly change. Another proverb says about people who are strong and swift that "time and unexpected events overtake them all." A car accident, a slip trip or fall, a heavy object falling on us, we can be victim of a crime, a natural disaster etc. The list is endless. We can suddenly and unexpectedly, be dealing with an old age injury or disease. So, wisdom would have us look ahead and view having a Hydrogen Water Therapy System now like a health insurance policy for our future.

Drinking hydrogen water now would have our older bodies in a much stronger condition to endure a sudden injury or disease and potentially recover from it faster and more completely.

## How does a home hydrogen water system work?

There are two "systems" needed, both complementary to each other, that when properly matched, make a complete high-quality, home, high-tech, Hydrogen Water Therapy System.

First, we begin with a pre-ionizer purification system. The economical approach is to install a small point of delivery pre filter near the water ionizer. The pre-filter option needs at least a two-stage pre filter with the highest quality parts, best design and most effective medias used to remove "hard-to-remove" contaminants along with a filter cartridge that can "soften" the source water that is hard.

Why installing a quality pre filter is so important? This is because the source water is so toxic that ionizer filters alone simply cannot remove most of the toxins. If it were built to do so the ionizer housing would be two to three times larger would not fit under a sink and be too large for most countertops causing people to decline buying a water ionizer.

Secondly, we complete our Hydrogen Water Therapy System with the water ionizer that clearly has an innovative design which should be a certified medical device with its own advanced filtration cartridge that completes the purification process.

Source water enters the pre filter purification stage, and those hard-to-remove contaminants are trapped in the pre filter media. Next, the source water is softened. Only after these processes, the source water is well accepted and ready to enter a water ionizer. Before the water passes over titanium plates dipped or coated in platinum, it needs more advanced filtration. A high-quality ionizer will have filter(s) with advanced filtration designs through which the water passes just before entering the ionization chamber.

Water ionization is the miracle process by which Molecular Hydrogen is created. When water is made to pass over the platinum coated titanium plates housed inside an ionizing machine, and electricity is run, the process of electrolysis takes place.

Water gets split into two streams. One stream is alkaline, the primary "drinking water" for Hydrogen Water Therapy. The other stream is mildly to strongly acidic – the extremely useful waters – that can be used for many applications (detailed discussion on strongly acidic water is outside the scope of this book).

## The pH scale

Proper pH is a crucial factor in good health. The pH is logarithmic; meaning the difference in one pH unit is a difference of ten times. If any substance changes from pH 7.0 to pH 8.0, it becomes ten times more alkaline. Similarly, if the pH comes down from the neutral 7.0 pH to a pH of 6.0, it means it is ten times more acidic. For example, a soda pop (cold drinks and beverages) at pH 2.5 is almost 50,000 times more acidic than 7.0 pH neutral water.

Imagine drinking the healthy pH 9.5 alkaline water and then drink that same can of soda pop at having acidity of pH 2.5. This means ten million times more acidic.

Of course, our well-designed stomach digestive system can adjust to this anomaly occasionally. It is not suggested that one can of soda pop is going to kill you, but the above illustration should be obvious. A regular continued consumption of highly acidic beverages could and probably would negate most of the beneficial alkaline properties of Hydrogen Water.

The next benefit of drinking freshly ionized hydrogen alkaline water is that it contains millions of antioxidants. We need to flood our bodies with an abundance of antioxidants. We all are aware that excessive oxidation in our bodies is harmful. Oxidative stress when left to run wild inside your body for weeks, months or even years will often lead to serious health problems and diseases.

Hydrogen is unique among all antioxidants is that it is selective and does not interfere on neutralize the important reactive oxygen species

(ROS). The most effective, efficient, and expedient way to deliver this superior antioxidant is to provide our bodies the freshly made ionized water daily which is Alkaline and contains abundant Hydrogen as antioxidant in each glass of water we drink.

Antioxidants can be measured using an ORP meter. ORP stands for "oxidation reduction potential." Any (+) ORP readings are signs of oxidation and any (–) ORP readings denote anti-oxidation. Aging results in degeneration of organs, bones, muscles, tendons, and the cellular membranes. The physical effect is results in formation of wrinkles and hair loss. An antioxidant reducing agent is simply something that inhibits or slows the process of oxidation.

The (+) ORP of most tap waters is between (+) 100 mV to (+) 200 mV and so is an oxidizing agent. Most bottled waters are both acidic and have higher (+) ORP's, making them increase our internal oxidation. Sodas, sports, and energy drinks can be even worse. Some of these have acidic pH as low as pH 2.5 and are extremely oxidizing with (+) ORP readings as high as (+) 500 mV.

As per studies, the benefit of drinking hydrogen water is the amount of Molecular Hydrogen gas dissolved in it. The beneficial range is from 0.05 mg/L to 1.6 mg/L. A highly quality water ionizer should produce a therapeutic dose of 0.5 mg/L (0.5 ppm) to 1.6 mg/L (1.6 ppm) depending on its power setting or capacity in relation to its progressive alkaline levels.

Some choose to drink hydrogen water produced through water electrolysis, but many others use portable devices or products such as hydrogen generator or tablet that can add about 1.0 ppm, usually based on a 500 ml amount of water. But those portable devices or tablets do not filter the water. They can only make a therapeutic dose of hydrogen medical gas usually in about 5 minutes. Portable devices and products can never replace a complete Hydrogen Water Therapy System that has filter to remove hundreds of contaminants.

Is more Hydrogen better? Early studies appeared to say yes! And it also appears you cannot get too much Hydrogen this is because it does not build up in our bodies. We simply exhale any excess. So, in many cases, the more hydrogen the better! Of course, health benefits will vary widely from person to person and more research needs to be done.

## Many more good things about Hydrogen Water

- Drinking a therapeutic dose of hydrogen water via at least one glass, but preferably 500 ml results in a peak rise in plasma and blood concentration in as little as 5 to 15 minutes. Depending on dosage, return to baseline will be in 45 to 90 minutes.
- Early research shows that hydrogen has a residue an effect that continues improving health or disease symptoms up to 4 weeks.
- Drinking 1 to 2 glasses of Hydrogen water after sleeping for 6 to 8 hours replenishes our body's reserve and primes our digestive tract for breakfast.
- Drinking one or two glasses before a main meal curbs our tendency to overeat. When water is consumed before a meal we tend to chew more completely, rather than washing food down.
- Hydrogen water is a perfect delivery fluid when talking nutritional supplements. It can ensure maximum absorption.

*"Hydrogen Water Therapy System"*

*- the need of every household*

Please refer to the following link, where global doctors and scientists have shared some human studies:

www.molecularhydrogeninstitute.com

Click on Research:
- Articles
- Scientific Studies

> *"Hydrogen Water Therapy System"*
>
> *- a Single Premium Lifetime Health Insurance for the entire family.*

# HYDRATION AND PERMEABILITY WITH STRUCTURED ELECTROLYZED REDUCED WATER

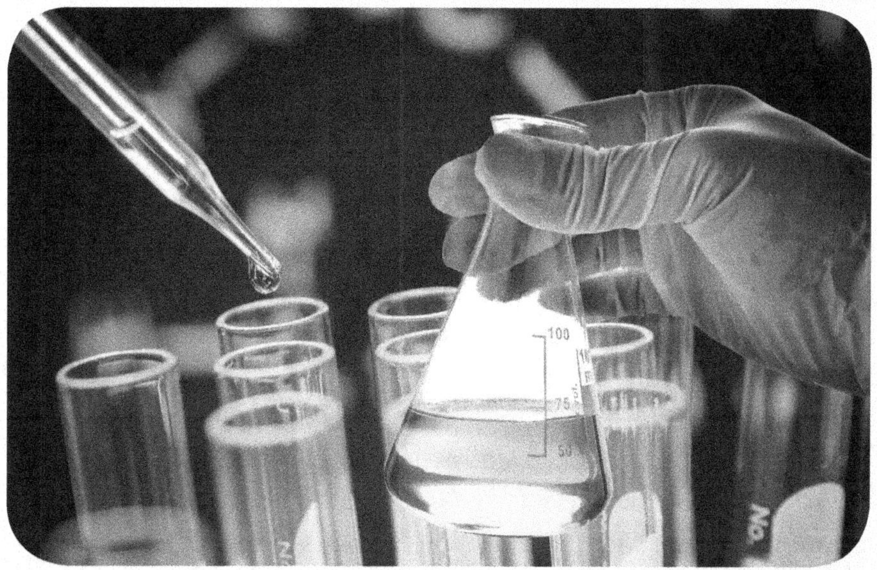

Why is it that some healing protocols have a lot of success than the others? Why is it some protocols that are extremely successful, you have never heard of?

The people who drank the structured water survived the Chernobyl Radiation Poisoning. The following is that incident which is available on the Internet.

On April 26, 1986, there was a nuclear meltdown of reactor No# 4 in Chernobyl, Ukraine. This is the most severe nuclear disaster in the history by far. Massive amounts of radiation were released into the atmosphere and spread over an enormous area by prevailing wind currents and a huge population was severely affected.

After initially denying that there was any problem, the government evacuated more than a lakh people from 7,50,000-acre area surrounding the site of the disaster. Most of these people had suffered immense radiation exposure prior to their evacuation. Many more people in areas well outside of the evacuation zone also suffered strong radiation exposure. Many thousands ultimately died of radiation poisoning.

In the years following this disastrous nuclear accident, an anomalous occurrence was discovered. The people living in a remote Caucasus Mountain region, which had been blanketed by radiation, were somehow spared the expected effect which had been observed in surrounding areas. This region was well known for its healing springs. Miraculously, in the village where the springs were located, nobody had contracted cancer or radiation sickness. This was quite unexplainable.

A team of top Russian scientists let by Dr. Igor Smirnov was sent to the area to investigate this. The scientists studied all the potential factors to try to explain the anomalous results. At first nothing could be identified. Finally, an investigation of the water everybody drank was conducted. There was nothing unusual identified in the water's mineral or chemical content. But, as they looked deeper, they discovered that the arrangement of the molecules in their drinking water was most unusual.

The mountain spring water was found to be unique in its structure and action on account of the geomagnetic field. The water got rapidly penetrated and efficiently absorbed into the bodies of the locals who were affected by the catastrophic radiation. The harmful effects of radiation to the body cells were therefore nullified prior to any damage.

Water molecules are usually bound together in a random fashion and form large loosely arranged clusters. For cells of the human body to absorb ordinary water molecules and become hydrated, the body must expend a lot of energy to break apart the clusters. However, when water is structured, i.e., organized as single individual molecules or as a chain of individual molecules, it can readily slip into the cells of the human body.

The special water of this region was naturally structured and could very efficiently and totally hydrate human cells with which it came into contact. This contrasts with the large, clustered form of water molecules that exists in most sources of water.

The water that the people living in the Caucasus Mountain region (lying between black sea and Caspian Sea and occupied by Russia, Georgia, Azerbaijan, and Armenia) were drinking – was inherently structured. As a result, the cells in the bodies of this population were being efficiently flushed and cleansed. The radioactive toxins stood no chance of persisting in this group of people.

They were just drinking this structured water which was allowing them to hydrate. Dr. Peter Agre was awarded with a Nobel Prize in 2003 for discovering "Aquaporins." There are these openings that are only few molecules of water wide in every cell. As per Dr. Agre, the "Aquaporins" form the plumbing system for the cells. Every human cell is primarily water. Aquaporins (the water channels, which are integral membrane pore proteins) selectively conduct water molecules in and out of the cell, while preventing the passage of ions and other solutes.

In a hydrated cell viruses are not able to multiply. So, if we give the body what it needs to function optimally, we can avoid the life-threatening protocols involving chemotherapy, radiation, and drugs.

It is not the cancer that really hurts people. Statistically around 45% of the patients having cancer will die of cachexia, meaning wasting of protein – all their lean body mass. The rest of them, then, die from the treatment.

When a patient gets immune-suppressed and they have cancer, what takes them? Liver failure, kidney failure, pneumonia, sepsis – but all these things are usually associated with also the person getting chemo and radiation.

The main reason for proper hydration of cells is that the water molecules go inside through these openings or channels one by one with the speed of several billion per second.

The human body must re-organize the water in "single linear structure" for penetration inside the cells easily. If the water has different type of structure or if it is densely clustered, which we generally consume, it requires a lot of energy for the human body to create proper structure.

Every part of the body is dependent on water. It is the foundation of all life on planet earth. The functions of our glands and organs will deteriorate if they are not nourished with clean water. Metabolism, blood flow and our cellular reproduction is dependent on proper absorption of water which is an excellent solvent.

If your body is not properly hydrated, the cells will draw water from your bloodstream, which will cause your heart to work harder. The kidneys also start to malfunction, and blood is not purified properly. This results in some of the kidney's workload to be passed on to the liver and other organs, which can cause them to be stressed.

Additionally, quite several minor health challenges can crop up, such as constipation, dry and itchy skin, acne, nosebleeds, urinary tract infection, coughs, sneezing, sinus pressure, and headaches.

To help our in-built Immune system to protect us from the daily hazards that we face daily, we need to support it by drinking structured water. This will ensure that our bodies are protected on an ongoing basis by receive adequate hydration.

Switch to Electrolyzed Reduced Water and start feeling the difference right away. You shall feel the difference inside out.

# ROLE OF ELECTROLYZED REDUCED WATER IN STOPPING THE FREE RADICAL CYCLE OF OXIDATION

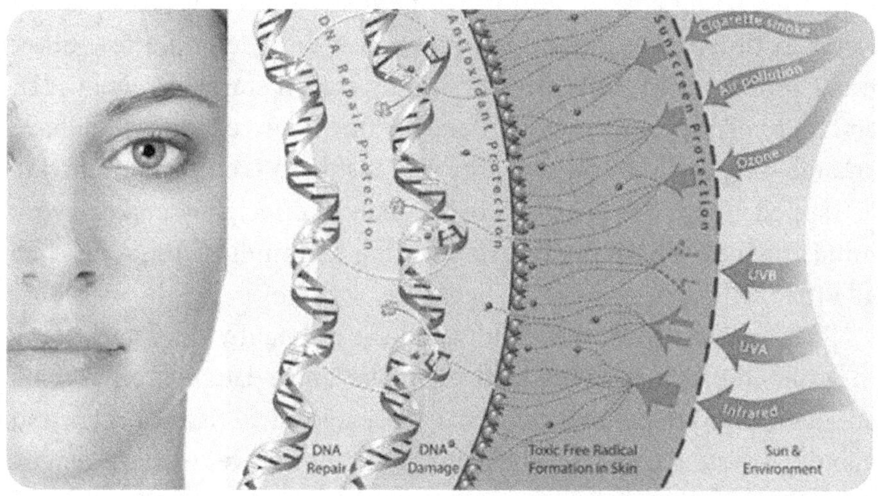


Oxidation happens when free radicals bombard our cells. We have about 30 trillion cells in our body and every day each one of these cells is assaulted by more than 10,000 free radicals. That damage is called oxidation. Free radicals are just atoms or molecules that have lost an electron. This can happen with exposure to UV radiation or lights. Hazards include things like fluorescent light bulbs, smoking, computers, cell phones, air travel, cars and many plants, fertilizers, and pesticides. Free radicals are also there in our drinking water and the air we breathe.

All those 30 trillion cells all have few things in common: fat being one of them. These cells all have membranes, and they are called the "Phospholipids Bilayer." Fat is one of the things that are the most easily oxidized substances in our body. We can see examples of that in our own kitchen. If we have ever fried anything then later, we try to clean that vent fan and that fat is thick and sticky. That is oxidized fat.

Our cell membranes are made primarily out of fat and as these are free radicals in our bodies, they start stealing electrons from the fat causing a huge problem. That fat then changes its character. Primarily, being a semi permeable membrane, it allows oxygen and water to flow freely in, and letting carbon dioxide and a few other waste products out. But instead of doing that, it starts to repel water, and the cell becomes dehydrated. So now the cell does not have enough oxygen to produce energy and inside the cell carbon dioxide is trapped along with other waste products. It effectively makes a very unhealthy cell. These then starts dividing and multiplying – just like all other cells do.

So effectively, both the healthy and the unhealthy cells start doing the same thing. They get divided and make 2 new daughter cells which are identical to the parent cell. This process leads to tissue, organ, and glandular system changes within our bodies. Wherever we have genetic weakness is in our body, whether it is in eyes, our heart or our blood vessels or our skin or our pancreas; the illness or the disease process is going to manifest wherever that weakness link is.

We all know about antioxidants. We know that Vitamins A, C and E are antioxidants. We know that all the brightly colored fruits and vegetables, even chocolates and coffee contain antioxidants. In theory the more antioxidants we consume, the more reversal of oxidation in your body or the more it will stop that free radical damage.

But there is a little-known fact about these antioxidants that we take in supplement form or in our foods. They make the free radical ineffective but by becoming a weak free radical. So, it donates an electron to a "Really Bad" free radical and in turn becomes a "Weak" free radical itself.

These supplements can therefore slow down the process of ageing, disease, and death to certain extent, but it cannot never really make a big enough impact to stop or reverse it.

People report positive changes in their health after taking Electrolyzed Reduced Water produced through the Ionization process as it is capable of dramatically reducing the rates of oxidation on their cells. When this happens, the body starts coming back to healthier states. We have all along been focusing on the wrong things all the time.

"Hydrogen and fuel cell technology (HFCT)" uses fuel cells to convert the stored chemical energy in hydrogen into electrical energy. Hydrogen is the simplest element and the most plentiful gas in the Universe. Just like this HFCT, the water ($H_2O$) when passed through an electric field gets split and becomes $OH^-$ and $H^+$. So, we have Hydrogen and in the presence of Platinum, which exists in all Hydrogen Fuel Cells and this Hydrogen easily and freely give up its electrons.

So now what do we have? We have a bunch of free electrons. In HFCT those free electrons are put down as a wire and you get electricity. In ionized water, these free electrons are recycled into the water. So, as we drink that water, we are taking in a bunch of free electrons. Now those free electrons will go and mitigate or quench the free radicals playing havoc in your body and they do not leave anything in their wake. There is no weak free radical leftover.

## Oxidation Reduction Potential (ORP)

We can measure an antioxidant's potential to supply electrons dispersed into a liquid by using an ORP (Oxidation/Reduction Potential) meter. Oxidized materials are shown as +above zero, antioxidants are either a low+ or a negative reading. Lower numbers indicate more available electrons. For example, the antioxidant CoQ10 (Coenzyme Q10) has an ORP of around (+) 50mV and Wheatgrass juice has an ORP of (-) 120mV. The negative reading of Wheatgrass juice gives a higher potential for putting electrons and neutralizing free radicals than CoQ10.

Electrolyzed Reduced Water is the most powerful Antioxidant with high Oxidation Reduction Potential to protect and heal and this inhibits the Cycle of Oxidation.

Electrolyzed Reduced Water protects our tissues, spinal cord, and the joints. It not only quenches our thirst and regulates our body's temperature but keeps the tissues in our body wet. We know how it feels when our eyes, nose or mouth gets dry; Right? The simplest way to maintain optimum levels of moisture in all the above sensitive areas, as well as in the blood, bones and brain is to keep ourselves hydrated adequately. Water also helps to protect the spinal cord, as well as acts as a lubricant in our joints.

I personally drink 8-10 glasses water from my ionizer with the pH setting at 9.5 and provides ORP of about (-) 400 mV.

The reality of the power of Electrolyzed Reduced Water is… JUST DRINK THE WATER! You will start feeling the difference almost immediately.

# ELECTROLYZED REDUCED WATER FOR GUT HEALTH AND LONGEVITY

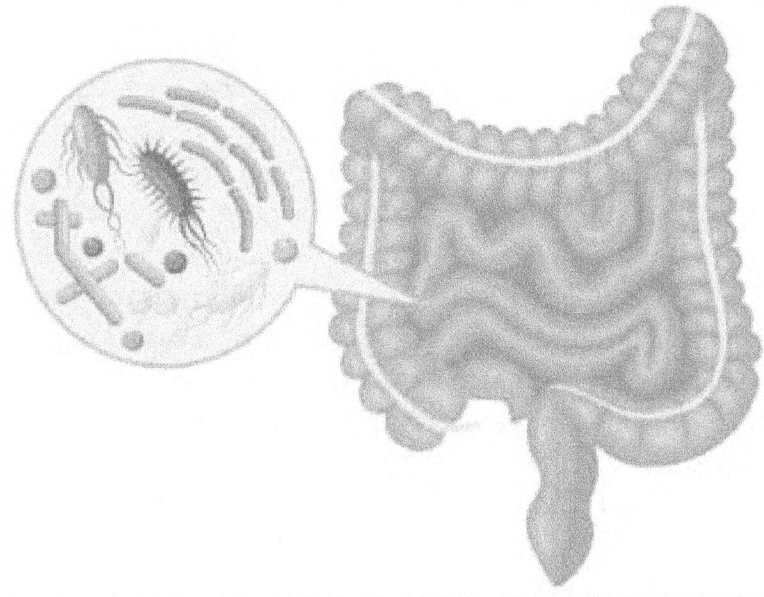

I had a lot of health issues, especially chronic irritable bowel syndrome for more than 30 years and tried so many streams of conventional treatments. Invariably the problems used to strike back with vengeance.

But when I tried Hydrogen rich Electrolyzed Reduced Water for approximately 3 months at a stretch now for more than 6 years, I could not figure out how it worked; it not only worked but worked so well in such a short span of time. This water completely changed my life – I feel like a new man. I now have more energy for workout, and have the motivation to eat better, which helped me manage the

IBS issue to a tolerable extent for which I have struggled with for decades!

I have a perfect BMI now and do not suffer from any lifestyle related or chronic disorders. And I have my latest diagnostic test reports to validate my claims. I firmly believe that this water has played its role in this transformation along with "Homeopathic Nosodes." It is not that I do not have health challenges. But they are far from few and not chronic and quite manageable with diet changes, exercise and meditation and keeping away from the ill effects of the mainstream media. I need to extend deepest gratitude to my Homeopathic Doctor who is also a big supporter of this Water Therapy.

The key to supporting me in my IBS issue might well be the power of the Electrolyzed Reduced Water. In this quest of getting to understand the healing properties of this water, I started my online extensive studies. I also started getting testimonies of people who also have been benefitted immensely with this water for a variety of their health issues.

Narrated below is a summary of my understanding on a very interesting topic on "Gut Microbiome" – which might be the key to our digestive issues.

## Health Begins in the "Gut – the Invisible Organ"

Let me introduce you to one of the hottest topics in medicine today – the "Gut Microbiome" – the complex colonies of microbial life within us. You can think of this as a new organ which you have just discovered. It relates to all other organs in the body.

It regulates immunity, our overall health and mental state – and the best part is that we are now learning to understand and work with it!

Autoimmune Diseases, Obesity, Diabetes, Irritable Bowel Syndrome, Autism, Parkinson's... the list goes on. For them, hope arrived with fixing the Microbiome. It is our very own internal ecosystem of beneficial bacteria, fungi, and viruses… all working together to fight disease and keep us healthy.

There are hundreds and trillions of microbes that are within our gut microbiome and that broad array includes some friendly bacteria which helps us function well. We commonly talk about Lactobacillus and Bifidobacteria but there are other bacteria that are unfriendly where it can be quite harmful if they get out of control.

People hear about Clostridium Difficile as a potential microbe that could harm us or E. coli from food borne outbreaks in fruits, vegetables, and meat. So, these are things that can actually be within our bodies or our gut microbiome and these we call pathogens are the microbes that can actually hurt us. Most of the times we have them in very low quantities and are outnumbered by the friendly ones and they are kept in check and in good balance.

Studies say that certain bacteria, the anaerobes, move best in negative ORP (oxidation reduction potential) and this is exactly that is made available by consistent use of ionized drinking water (the antioxidant value of high alkaline water is represented by this ORP measurement).

It allows for the growth of protective microflora, (mostly) the lactic acid bacteria such as Lactobacilli and Bifidobacteria. These bacteria guard against overgrowth of gram negative, toxin-producing aerobes.

The produced toxin growth of the aerobes is also important to health, but never should they be overgrown in the small intestine as it leads to a mal-absorption syndrome and is associated with metabolic diseases such as diabetes, obesity, cancer, and neurodegenerative diseases.

Creating an ideal environment by drinking high negative-value (ORP) drinking water – which is the high alkaline water, the protective microbe in our intestinal fort is guarded.

## The Protective Power of the Gut Microbiota which gets raised with High Alkaline Water!

There is a reciprocal relationship that we have with our own microbes. We need a healthy balance of our gut microbiota for our health and survival. This field of Microbiome has been exploding with the latest findings and research. It is possible to make a true paradigm shift in health and medicine based on the findings.

Drinking high negative-value ORP drinking water is all about a health mechanism of maintaining an environment by which our protective microbiota thrives. The environment is that of our small intestines where the maximum amount of water gets absorbed.

The small intestine may be treated as the center of all health; it is here where there is a balance to balance the microbes. This is where our nutrients are absorbed or mal-absorbed. This is where all health begins, or it may become the beginning of the end!

There is a general conception that drinking high alkaline water is harmful as it would make our intestines more alkaline. But it is the opposite. Drinking high alkaline water favors the growth of microbes which maintain the intestinal pH at healthy acidic levels.

To re-phrase the popular belief, the so-called alkaline diet is the one that feeds the protective microbiota to maintain a healthy acidic gut. A low acid gut means acid reflux, and to cure it the acid must be raised. When there is an acid production in the gut, bicarbonate is sent into circulation to maintain healthy alkaline blood. Can you understand the inverse relationships of our compartmentalized bodies? These inverse relationships include gut-brain and intracellular pH and everything starts in the gut where our water is absorbed.

Therefore, by creating an alkaline environment with a high negative-value of ORP drinking water, we are assisting our protective microbes to flourish thereby helping the intestinal terrain to remain active.

Healthy acidic gut is created by high alkaline water. The Research article links are given below for you to supplement your quest for further explanations.

**"Food & Hydration Version 1.0" was all about SURVIVAL**. If your intake consists of a good number of calories to fill your stomach and drink any beverage to take care of your thirst mechanism – then that is great, and it has been the reality for most of human history.

In this modern era, we are dominated by **"Food & Hydration Version 2.0" where the goal is COMMERCE.** This system unfortunately is morally bankrupt as it has delivered a food and beverage system mostly devoid of nutrients but packed with junk, toxins, and sugar.

We now need **"Food & Hydration Version 3.0," where the central organizing principle is HEALTH, Health for our BODIES and Health for our PLANET.** There are plenty of healthy profits to be made (and to flourish), in this version as well.

Drinking Ionized, Structured, Alkalized Water with High Oxidation Reduction Potential (ORP) may be the simplest and least expensive way to regain health and enjoy life with energy, mental clarity, peace, equanimity, and comfort.

Treat yourself and your family members with "Alkaline Ionized Water with abundant Molecular Hydrogen" created with the most advanced water systems in the world.

*So, Feed Your Microbes... Nurture Your Mind!!*

<u>Visit:</u>
https://www.sciencedaily.com/releases/2016/09/160916114635.htm

*Positive Effect of on Electrolyzed Reduced Water on Gut Permeability, Fecal Microbiota and Liver in an Animal Model of Parkinson's Disease.*

Visit for more: **https://pubmed.ncbi.nlm.nih.gov/31600256/**

Read the full article here:
**https://journals.plos.org/plosone/article?id=10.1371/journal.pone.0223238**

*"A clinical study shows that the negative ORP of ERW creates a gut environment by which protective microbiota, especially anaerobic bacteria, thrives allowing a protection against pathogenic bacteria in patients with irritable bowel syndrome."*

**https://pubmed.ncbi.nlm.nih.gov/29849734/**

*Effects of Alkaline-Reduced Drinking Water on Irritable Bowel Syndrome with Diarrhea: A Randomized Double-Blind, Placebo-Controlled Pilot Study*

Visit: **https://www.hindawi.com/journals/ecam/2018/9147914/**

"Microorganisms have their own intrinsic reduction potential (Eh) for each species, and aerobic and anaerobic bacteria grow at different oxidation-reduction potentials. Aerobic bacteria require a positive potential of (+) 400 mV and facultative anaerobic bacteria require negative electric potential between (−) 300 and (−) 400 mV.

Electrochemically generated reduced water has a negative potential of 0 to (−) 300 mV, while the tap water has a potential of (+) 300 to (+) 450 mV. By drinking reduced water, it is possible to improve symptoms of functional bowel disease by accelerating the growth of anaerobic bacteria (Lactobacilli and Bifidobacteria) and inhibiting the growth of aerobic pathogens." (2018)

**https://www.sciencedirect.com/science/article/abs/pii/ S030698770400489X**

# THE ROLE OF MOLECULAR HYDROGEN IN ACTIVATION OF NRF2 – THE HEAD OF OUR INTERNAL DEFENSE SYSTEM

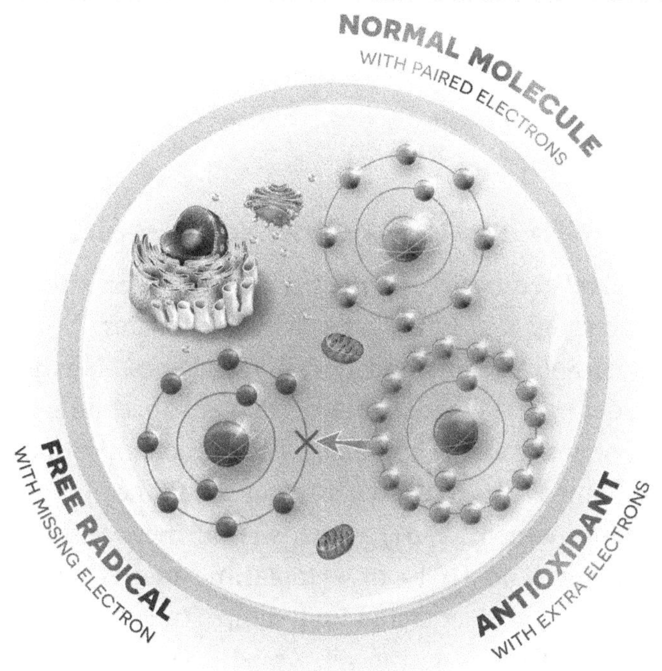



(Chapter Acknowledgement: https://drjockers.com/nrf2-benefits/)

Oxidative stress is one of the major players in the formation of pathological conditions such as cancer, diabetes, and heart disease, which also accelerates aging and neurodegeneration. Antioxidant rich foods, herbs and supplements are there to protect the body from unwanted oxidative stress. Recent research has found a new signaling pathway that plays an enormous role in amplifying the effects of antioxidants on the body.

The body adapts to function in a state of homeostasis or balance. When the body faces major stressors, the cells should quickly modulate their antioxidant capacity to counteract the increased oxidative stress. To do this, the body should be capable of activating a massive antioxidant effect in a matter of few nanoseconds through a specific genetic pathway.

In this chapter, you will discover ways to activate the antioxidant benefits of the NRF2 gene pathway.

## The Keap1-NRF2 Pathway and Your Health

NRF2 (NF E2 related factor 2) is a transcription factor among humans that is encoded by a specific gene, which regulates the expression of a bunch of antioxidants and detoxifying genes. This pathway is activated under times of oxidative stress that enhance the expression of a multitude of antioxidants and phase II liver detoxification enzymes that restore homeostasis to the ox/redox cycles in the body.

An enzyme (named Keap1) which sits on the cytosol of the cell [the intracellular fluid (ICF) or cytoplasmic matrix], is the liquid found inside cells. It is separated into compartments by membranes, interacts with NRF2 and activates it. Keap1 is rich in the amino acid: cysteine, and acts as a sensor that constantly reads the environment for any increase or decrease in oxidative stress. In times of increased oxidative stress, Keap1 activates NRF2 which then migrates into the cell nucleus and merges with the DNA to activate the Antioxidant Response Element (ARE). ARE then regulates a variety of powerful antioxidant enzymes and detoxifying proteins.

This Keap 1 NRF2 pathway regulates over 600 genes involved in cellular protection and antioxidant defenses. These different genes act as a booster to major antioxidant and detoxifying enzymes such as glutathione and superoxide dismutase. They also help in improving tissue healing and repairs and assist in anti-inflammatory prostaglandins and enzymes.

The most common NRF2 activators known are Curcumin (from turmeric spice). This along with Resveratrol (available in grapes), Quercetin (we get from Onions) and Sulforaphane (available in broccoli) activate NRF2 by different mechanisms when taken together, may be synergistic, or more effective when separated.

We can get remarkable health benefits by supplementing with NRF2 activators. These include reducing inflammation and pain, reducing insulin resistance and protection against a host of degenerative and immune-based diseases.

To better understand the role of NRF2, one needs to have a basic knowledge of Free Radicals, Antioxidants and Food Supplements.

## What are Free Radicals?

Free radicals are the ones that damage the growth, survival, and development of cells in the body. Their reactive nature allows them to engage in unnecessary side reactions that cause cellular impairment and eventually injury when they are present in disproportionate amounts. They directly impair cell membranes and DNA.

A molecule with one or more unpaired electrons in the outer shell is called a free radical. Free radicals are formed from molecules through the breakage of a chemical bond, that each fragment keeps one electron, by cleavage of a radical to give another radical and, also via redox reactions. Please refer to the link for details:

**https://www.ncbi.nlm.nih.gov/pmc/articles/PMC3614697/**

Free radicals, as well as unstable molecules with unpaired electrons, are an unavoidable byproduct of cellular metabolism. By stealing electrons from lipids, proteins, RNA and DNA, the free radicals cause damage to them.

Atoms are surrounded by electrons that orbit the atom in layers and those are called shells. Each shell must be filled with a set number of electrons. When a shell is full, electrons begin filling up the next shell. An atom whose outer shell is not full may bond with another atom using their electrons to complete its own outer shell. These are free radicals and are unstable. Atoms with a full outer shell are considered stable.

When oxygen molecules separate themselves into single atoms that consist of unpaired electrons, they try to steal other atoms or molecules to bond it with others. This instability is free radical formation which is the start of oxidative stress.

These are so dangerous that they even try to take away the proteins and the lipids of your tissues. These then become damaged, dysfunctional and are not capable of fulfilling their roles. Free radicals are the byproduct of the ordinary energy-producing processes. They are produced deep within the cells and are thought to be responsible for aging and disease, including even cancer.

## How are Free Radicals formed?

Free radicals get created by mental stress, which is due to steroid hormone cortisone, produced by the adrenal cortex. Also, the cells and tissues of different systems of our bodies secrete catecholamine. Free radicals are a byproduct of cell metabolism. Free radicals get generated from the food we eat, the air we breathe and the water we drink. It is results from the medicines we take, alcohol, tobacco, smoke, pesticides, and air pollutants to name a few.

## How do free radicals damage the body?

Various studies and theories have connected oxidative stress due to accumulation of free radical damage to:

- Central nervous system diseases, such as Alzheimer's and other dementias.
- Cardiovascular disease due to clogged arteries.
- Autoimmune and inflammatory disorders, such as rheumatoid arthritis and cancer.
- Cataracts and age-related vision decline.
- Age-related changes in appearance, such as loss of skin elasticity, wrinkles, graying hair, hair loss, and changes in hair texture.
- Diabetes.
- Genetic degenerative diseases, such as Huntington's disease or Parkinson's.

## What are Antioxidants?

The antioxidants are those compounds that are capable to inhibit oxidation; they are substances that may protect your cells against free radicals.

Examples of antioxidants include Vitamins C and E, Selenium and Carotenoids, such as beta-carotene, lycopene, lutein, and zeaxanthin (one of the most common carotenoid alcohols found in nature).

Foods that are high in antioxidants include – Broccoli, Spinach, Carrots, and potatoes. Also included in this list are Artichokes, Cabbage, Asparagus, Avocados, Beetroot, Radish, Lettuce, Sweet Potatoes, Squash, Pumpkin, Collard Greens, and Kale. We must use lots of spices which are available abundantly in our food preparations.

## Dietary Supplementation

We first need to ascertain if an individual is already consuming an ideal diet or not. If the answer is no, then there is a potential benefit. The question then becomes what supplements are best to provide nutrients that are most likely to be sub-optimal in your diet.

Based on current theories in nutrition, our diets should have plenty of vegetables included (especially raw) and fruit. But most people probably do not get optimal amounts of the nutrients (vitamins, minerals, antioxidants, trace elements) associated with these vegetables and fruits.

"Oxidative Stress" leads to a host of disease which includes diabetes, hypertension, cardiovascular diseases, obesity, arthritis, liver disease and some cancers. The nutritional research supports this belief. Oxidative Stress is an abundance of reactive oxygen species (ROS), or "free radicals", that are destructive molecules in our food and our environment. Our cells have in-built protective mechanisms to fight these ROS. They manufacture antioxidants that can neutralize ROS, but as we age there is a gradual impairment of these systems resulting in less antioxidant activity thus greater damage to our DNA, RNA and cells which impairs function and can lead to the above diseases.

Since long, science has validated the use of antioxidants to promote optimal health as they could offset the damages of oxidative stress. The use of antioxidants is widespread and food supplements are widely recommended. Studies showed diets that are high in natural antioxidants [such as the Mediterranean (anti-inflammatory) diet, Okinawan, or Paleo diets] – they all seem to provide protection against oxidative stress. Statistics suggest that populations following these diets have the less degenerative disease and greater longevity.

Normally, the antioxidants can neutralize the free radicals. They do this by gulping down the electrons from the free radicals, which renders the free radicals inert. The body has its own defense system against free radicals, the free radical detoxifying enzymes, and antioxidant chemicals. But when the free radicals are disproportionate to the antioxidant defenses; when the antioxidant defenses are outnumbered by hoards of free radicals, bad things happen.

For eliminating pathogens, short-term oxidative stress can be helpful. Free radicals are essential to life. The body's ability to turn air and food into chemical energy depends on a chain reaction of free radicals. Free radicals are also a crucial part of the immune system, floating through the veins and attacking foreign invaders.

It is when the free radicals get out of control that things go downhill.

So based on the above discussion, we have now understood that antioxidants help protect the body from oxidative stress. We have also learned that there are various antioxidants and supplements which help us overcome free radical bombardment.

## NRF2 – the Master Regulator of Anti-Oxidative Responses

**https://www.ncbi.nlm.nih.gov/pmc/articles/PMC5751370/**

Our bodies are continually bombarded by destructive molecules called free radicals which are like the chemical reaction that causes iron to rust. When these free radical toxins outnumber their counterbalance, which are the naturally produced antioxidants, it all leads to a condition known as oxidative stress which we all have.

Like the rusting of an engine, oxidative stress is not good for our bodies. This might be an explanation to the untimely motor neuron cell death as seen in Amyotrophic Lateral Sclerosis (ALS). This disease of the nervous system weakens the muscles and physical abilities get impaired. The cause of this disease is unknown. There is no cure of ALS but its progression can be slowed down by medication and therapy.

Oxidative stress is important in the pathophysiology of ALS. Some ALS patients lack the antioxidant enzyme, the superoxide dismutase, type 1 (SOD1) that naturally eliminates free radicals inside our cells.

When we take the foods or supplements having NRF2 activators, they can reduce the oxidative stress significantly by activating the NRF2 pathway within our cells.

NRF2 is... basically like a thermostat and works the same way as an air conditioner with a thermostat does. Instead of controlling temperature, NRF2 regulates the oxidative stress levels.

The body's built-in cellular protection system gets managed and regulated with NRF2. The NRF2 is turned on within the cell when the stress is high; it is turned off when the stress levels are low. It is on account this that the NRF2 protein is termed as the "master regulator" of antioxidants.

## NRF2 and Cancer Prevention

High levels of oxidative stress damage normal cells, affecting the DNA and inducing cancer causing mutations. Oxidative stress also creates chronic inflammatory pathways that favor an optimal environment for development and progression of cancer. Activation of the Keap1-NRF2 pathway has been shown to be productive against tumor formation.

## NRF2 and Brain Health

Globally, we now have an epidemic of neurodegenerative disorders. The Keap1-NRF2-ARE pathway has been researched to be a key player in the development or prevention of neurodegeneration.

Chronic inflammation is the cause of mood disorders such as depression, bipolar, addictions etc. The NRF2 pathway has been researched to come out as a major factor in the development of mood disorders and poor neurotransmitter function.

## NRF2 and Diabetes Prevention

Type II diabetes is characterized by chronic inflammation and oxidative stress. The major cause of chronic kidney disease and peripheral neuropathy is Diabetes. It is also one of the major factors leading to cardiovascular disease.

Research has indicated that the NRF2 pathway is reduced in type II diabetes as well as associated with hyperglycemia. The heavy formation of advanced glycolytic end products provokes tissue damage.

Research has indicated that having stability in the Keap1 and NRF2 pathway is crucial to the prevention of type II diabetes. Activating the Keap1 and NRF2 pathway also protects the body against the tremendous metabolic stress that diabetes creates. This also helps to stabilize blood sugar levels and reverse this disorder to some extent.

## NRF2 and Auto-Immunity

The Keap1-NRF2 pathway plays an important role in proper immune coordination. Studies that observed NRF2 deficient mice showed a great risk of developing autoimmune disorders. These include lupus, multiple sclerosis, rheumatoid arthritis, and others.

NRF2 deficient mice developed normal body structures but displayed a variety of autoimmune disorders and a shortened lifespan. The decreased glutathione production from the NRF2 deficient mice leads to immune mal-coordination and hyper-inflammatory processes.

## NRF2 and Hormonal Health

Loss of progesterone among women and testosterone among men leads to high levels of physical and emotional stress. It accelerates the aging process. Depletion of these key hormones leads to a state of estrogen dominance which is one of the major factors associated with degenerative disease processes. This is also the cause of menstrual and menopause issues in women.

The Keap1-NRF2 pathway regulates the expression of antioxidant enzymes such as glutathione peroxidase and NAD(P)H-quinone oxidoreductase 1 that helps remove toxic estrogen metabolites.

Estrogen is a growth factor and stimulates growth patterns in many forms of uterine, breast, cervical, ovarian, colon and prostate cancers. Research says that activation of the NRF2 pathway inhibits the estrogen signaling pathway in different forms of breast cancer.

## The NRF2 Activators

**Now that we have established the importance of NRF2, where do we get it from?**

There are several compounds which can be found in nature and are ingested through specific foods and herbs that enhance the Keap1-NRF2 pathway. You can find these nutrients in turmeric (curcumin), resveratrol in grape skin and berries (stilbenes), green tea and dark chocolate (catechins) and cruciferous veggies (sulforaphane). It is advised to consume these compounds daily. This will keep our antioxidant defense systems in balance, reduce formation of diseases, improve the quality of aging and above all improve the quality of life.

The added benefit of consuming these ingredients together is that they have a synergetic effect that amplifies their effects on the Keap1-NRF2 pathway. The easiest way this is done is through the key supplements that are specifically designed to up regulate this pathway.

## NRF2 Supplements

Although oxidative stress by itself will activate NRF2, you can enhance the effect by using certain compounds. Please read the labels if you wish to know the compounds are there in the supplements you are taking. There are plenty of studies that have evidence suggesting the medicinal benefits of the herbal supplements.

But there is a catch!

Overdosing or over activating the NRF2 pathway can have serious side effects. Normally these occur to people who are naturally allergic to the herbal components included in the supplement. The side effects can be minor to serious.

If you experience any side-effects while taking a supplement, please seek medical attention immediately. It is always suggested to consult your health care provider before taking any new supplements.

You are encouraged to refer to go through the following link on "The Effects of Dietary Supplements that over activate the NRF2/ARE System:"

**https://pubmed.ncbi.nlm.nih.gov/31099320/**

Let me now discuss about one very effective supplement which is based on solid research and is also safe.

## Enter: Molecular Hydrogen

The supplements and food supplements might have potential side effects. These cannot be blanket recommendation as few of the people might get adverse effects. But unlike these, Molecular Hydrogen has none. These all makes it a very interesting topic for clinical and pharmaceutical research at the present. There have been several well-conducted trials suggesting that Molecular Hydrogen is completely safe and has the same benefits as the available products in the market containing NRF2 activators.

In addition, there is another hidden benefit to Molecular Hydrogen compared to the other NRF2 synergizers (which are herbal dietary supplements marketed with unsupported claims that they can treat several medical conditions).

But to understand this benefit, we will need to know **"The Dark Side of NRF2!"**

Too much of any good thing can be bad! Even though NRF2 activation is useful in many cases, having the NRF2 pathway turned on all the time can harm the body. If the concentrations are high, the antioxidants can:

- Act as pro-oxidants, thereby increasing oxidation.
- Protect dangerous cells (such as cancer cells) as well as healthy cells.

- Reduce the health benefits of exercise.
- Have unwanted side effects, such as nausea and headaches or even reach toxic levels.

The dark side of NRF2 is that mutated cells or cancer cells can use the mutated form of a protein called Keap1 to their advantage. It will form a shield (protective barrier), that would protect them from chemotherapeutic agents. The immune system will not be able to do anything about it.

So, if the Keap1-NRF2 pathway is mutated, it can make the tumor grow faster and become more resistant. The protein, Keap1, contains multiple sensors. If these sensors together with the receptor regions are activated, the body will release NRF2, and it will pass into the nucleus. There is a region in the nucleus called Antioxidant Response Element. Certain genes here have very important having antioxidant properties. NRF2 on entering the nucleus binds itself to this region.

Cancer may be the reason if the Keap1 protein is mutated. The NRF2 protein cannot protect the body from this mutated protein. Studies indicate that having the NRF2 pathway activated constantly can increase the chance of mortality, hypertension, and albuminuria (a sign of kidney disease).

This is the opposite of what we want!

Molecular Hydrogen is a selective NRF2 activator; it works only when the body needs. It is a preventive and therapeutic medical gas for various diseases. Follow the link below:

**https://www.ncbi.nlm.nih.gov/pmc/articles/PMC5731988/**

In other words: With Molecular Hydrogen, you get the benefits of NRF2 activation when you need it, and none of the side effects that come from prolonged activation when you do not want.

It is earnestly hoped that now you have a basic understanding of what NRF2 is and how to choose a safe and effective NRF2 supplement to improve the quality of your life.

One of the simplest ways to accelerate the NRF2 antioxidant defense pathways is simply by drinking Electrolyzed Reduced Water rich in Molecular Hydrogen produced through Water Electrolysis. I can assist you to own this amazing piece of technology which renders ordinary tap water into Electrolyzed Reduced Water which brings the body back to balance.

# HYDROGEN: THE SMALLEST MOLECULE HAVING LARGE IMPACT ON HUMAN HEALTH

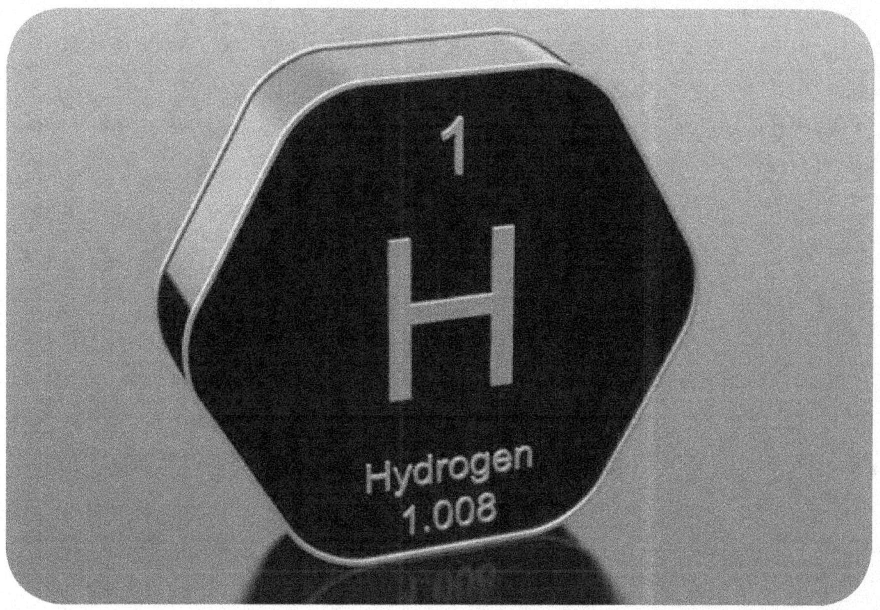

We either adapt to changes or we get left behind in an old, perhaps out-of-date, even high-risk approach to healthcare. Many global doctors and researchers believe hydrogen water therapy to be one of the greatest discoveries for a medical application in 67 years.

Molecular hydrogen gas is probably the greatest discovery in medical science and health care since 1953.

The DNA molecule structure was identified and mapped out by two scientists in 1953 who were awarded the Nobel Prize. Medical sciences were forever changed. When DNA was introduced, the sub-cellular world of nanotechnology, epigenetic came into light. We were introduced to the concept of personalized medicine.

Fast forward to 2005, Dr. Shigeo Ohta, Ph.D. makes a huge discovery. He declared that his entire life shall henceforth be devoted to developing the protective effects of the hydrogen gas for the humanity.

Today, it is a Global movement.

Hydrogen is two hydrogen atoms bonded together to form the lightest and smallest molecule of gas in our Universe. When infused into purified water, it produces a liquid that can hydrate virtually all of 37.2 trillion cells. This is done at a very fast speed at the epigenetic levels as seen under the microscope.

Therapeutic molecular hydrogen gas is not new to our planet. "Healing Springs" has been around for thousands of years. The chronically ill travel to these springs which exist in France, Mexico, India, Germany, Japan, and others to bathe and drink these waters. People often felt better, and their ailments disappeared. Recent research has confirmed that these waters contain dissolved hydrogen gas. Clinical studies and over 1,000 studies paper has demonstrated the marvel of this molecule for super health.

## How it Works

$H_2$ is an emerging medical gas therapy with unlimited potential to restore homeostasis to essentially every organ of our body. $H_2$ has potential to help with the top 8 out of 10 diseases causing fatalities.

- $H_2$ alters cell signaling, cell metabolism and gene expression, giving $H_2$ anti-inflammatory, anti-allergic, anti-obesity and anti-apoptotic (anti-cell death) effects.
- $H_2$ rapidly penetrates membranes to diffuse into our sub-cellular compartments, thus decreasing cytotoxic oxygen radicals, protecting our DNA, RNA, and proteins from oxidative stress.

- H$_2$ triggers activation or up-regulation of additional antioxidant enzymes throughout our body.
- As blood circulation increases by H$_2$, there are literally hundreds of benefits.

## Other benefits of H$_2$ gas

One benefit of H$_2$ is that it is very safe. Hundreds of studies prove its high safety profile. H$_2$ gas has been safely used for deep sea diving since the 1940s. Hydrogen is very natural to our body and is already present in our DNA and colon. And H$_2$ is non-radical, non-reactive, non-polar neutral gas with no noxious side effects.

Today the world of water is full of choices; Right?

We can choose old conventional out-of-date cheap water that attacks our bodies contributing or leading to over 90% disease… or… we can choose the new innovative, cutting-edge, ultra-pure H$_2$ water having science based anti-aging properties that can potentially protect the body from a plethora of elements and diseases.

> "It is an interesting parallel… that such a small; indeed, the smallest molecule can have a very large impact on human health."
>
> - Tyler LeBaron
> Molecular Hydrogen Institute /
> International Molecular Hydrogen Association.

One glass of water does not equal another. One may just pacify your thirst, while the other you may enjoy drinking; and in Japan, people know about this difference. And the whole world is now gradually getting aware of this phenomenon of availability of this water right in your home.

# Molecular Hydrogen – The Best Antioxidant for your Health

Antioxidants are a hot thing in the health and supplement universe today. Many of the supplement companies will claim that their antioxidant formulas are the best for your health, but none can really compare to the amazing properties of molecular hydrogen as best antioxidant to fight off oxidative stress.

The 3 properties that makes Molecular Hydrogen the best antioxidant ever:

## 1. Bioavailability (Size)

All together for antioxidants to be valuable, they must touch cell areas that have been harmed by dangerous free radicals. Generally, it is very difficult for the antioxidants to reach the mitochondria, where most free radicals are produced. What makes Molecular Hydrogen unique is its bioavailability.

Hydrogen is so small that it can penetrate through cells immediately and naturally being a gaseous state, using rapid diffusion and functions as a special antioxidant that is not blocked by normal mechanism that prevent other antioxidants from moving in our bodies.

Click here: **https://www.ncbi.nlm.nih.gov/pmc/articles/PMC325 7754/**

Hydrogen gas is the smallest and lightest particle comprising just two protons and two electrons. $H_2$ weighs 88 times less than Vitamin C which is the most famous antioxidant, and 215 times less than Coenzyme Q10 which is another prevalent cell reinforcement or antioxidant.

Hydrogen is likewise neutral and non-polar, enabling it to effortlessly go through the cells layers and sub-cellular compartments (mitochondria). It has a high dispersion rate which enables it to pervade cells easily.

## 2. It has Zero Toxicity (No unsafe by-products)

Unlike some antioxidants that can leave unsafe byproducts and create free radicals in the body, Molecular Hydrogen is considered one of the safest antioxidants for our bodies because it leaves no byproducts.

During the process of neutralizing the unsafe hydroxyl radicals by Hydrogen, it changes the form of the free radical to water which is advantageous to the body and does not require evacuation. Other antioxidants like Vitamin C for example can create Ascorbyl Radicals which are a natural indicator for oxidative stress[1,2].

## 3. Free Radical Selectivity

There are studies that show that not all free radicals are bad for the human body. But what makes Molecular Hydrogen such a special one as a selective antioxidant, is that it selectivity neutralizes the most cytotoxic (cells harming) free radicals, for example, the hydroxyl radical (OH).

**https://www.nature.com/articles/nm1577**

This is important because it allows our bodies to keep the free radicals that may be beneficial to while eliminating the free radicals that are truly damage our bodies.

## Medical Studies that backup Molecular Hydrogen ($H_2$)

Although Molecular Hydrogen is a new therapy it is backed by hundreds of studies in various backgrounds.

Click here to learn more: **http://www.molecularhydrogeninstitute. com/studies**

---

[1]  **https://www.hindawi.com/journals/bmri/2014/614506/**
[2]  **https://www.wikigenes.org/e/ref/e/7959177.html**

## Methods to take Molecular Hydrogen

### Molecular hydrogen Inhalation

You can breathe $H_2$ by attaching a facemask or nasal cannula to a molecular hydrogen gas generator gadget.

Breathing in Molecular Hydrogen gas acts more quickly than other techniques for consumption. So, it is a reasonable protection against intense (sudden) oxidative stress. (Stroke, Aggravation etc.) Molecular hydrogen gas inward breath has been utilized in doctor's facility settings under the care of social insurance specialists in Asia.

Although Molecular Hydrogen gas inward breath appears to have awesome advantages, it is unrealistic for regular utilization.

### Molecular hydrogen Saline Injection

Another technique for molecular hydrogen admission utilized in doctor's facility settings is the molecular hydrogen saline infusion.

A sack of saline (salt water) is imbued with molecular hydrogen gas which is then infused specifically into the circulation system of patients. This strategy is the most exact approach to quantify the measure of hydrogen that is directed to a patient. This strategy is famous in Japan where molecular hydrogen industry is the most developed. Molecular hydrogen is broadly perceived as a helpful particle and numerous items and administrations are based around molecular hydrogen. In any case, this technique is just suitable in clinical settings.

### $H_2$ Drinking Water

The most common method of consuming Hydrogen is drinking $H_2$ enriched water, simply called Hydrogen Water. Alkaline ionizer machines were the first sources of Hydrogen water (although at a lower concentrations).

## H$_2$ Supplements

H$_2$ supplements are the most effortless strategy to get Hydrogen into your body every day. Simply pop a couple of containers or tablets and high centralizations of Hydrogen will be delivered inside your stomach in almost no time.

But there are drawbacks with supplements which include:

- Hydrogen supplements use a chemical process to create Hydrogen unlike Hydrogen water generators that use an electrolysis process.
- Costs of using supplements over time can exceed Hydrogen water generators. So even though the upfront costs seem lower but over time it will potentially cost more.
- Also supplement pills have a shelf life so the efficacy of the supplement will diminish as time goes by.

## Hydrogen Bath

The Hydrogen bath will change your usual baths into a transdermal treatment by implanting your bath water with Hydrogen rich gas. The discharged air pockets moving against the body will be absorbed by the pores of the skin, breathed in through your lungs giving profound alleviating, beneficial medical advantages.

Numerous examinations have demonstrated advantages to Molecular Hydrogen treatment and now you can likewise appreciate reviving impacts of Hydrogen rich water in the solaces of your own home.

# COULD CORRECTING "VOLTAGE" BE THE ANSWER TO "CURING DISEASE"?

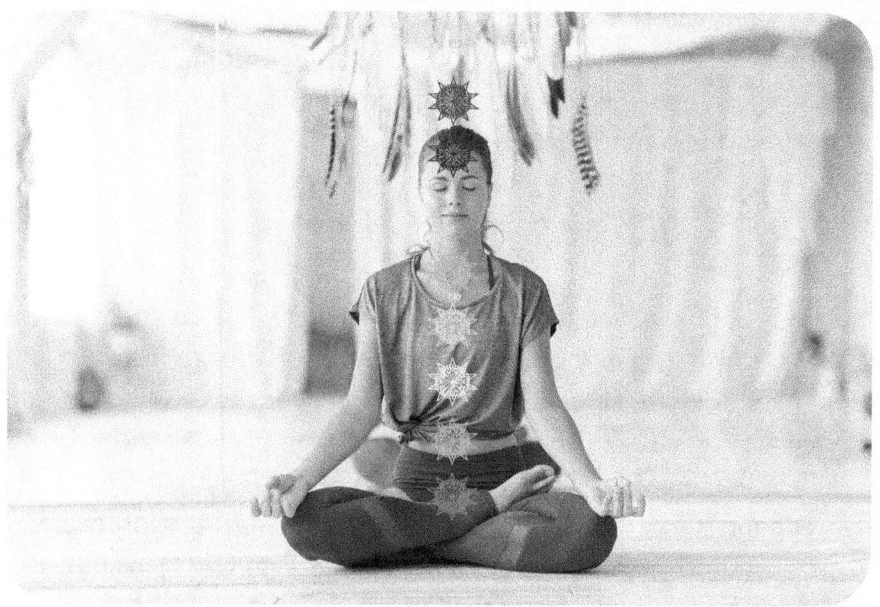

**(Chapter Acknowledgement: Dr. Jerry Tennant)**

The correct amount of voltage is needed to facilitate neurotransmission, cell repair, detoxification, and oxygenation/gas exchange. No activity occurs in your body without the presence of electrical charge.

We could say that there will be no life if there is no voltage. We can go a step further by stating, Low Voltage = Disease.

Research work done for over the last 100 years has shown for sure that the human cells which are healthy, operates at a voltage of (-) 25 mV. If new cells are to be made or a damaged cell needs to be repaired, the voltage needs to be increased to (-) 50 mV. For this process to happen there must be availability of all the nutrients required as well as proper and fast elimination of all things that damage the cells. The supply of voltage is totally dependent on the alkalinity and the pH (potential hydrogen) or the acid/alkaline balance.

To understand voltage in the body, one must understand the term **"pH"**. When you think about voltage in a copper wire, the switch is either on or off and electrons are either moving through the wire or not. However, in a liquid, you have the possibility of the solution to be an electron donor or an electron stealer.



It is a way of talking about the quantum of acid and base in our bodies. It is also a way of talking about the amount of voltage in our body. pH is measured on a logarithmic scale where 0 is the most acidic and fourteen (14) is alkaline to the maximum. Seven (7) is neutral.

When the ionization happens, water ($H_2O$) gets split into Hydrogen ($H^+$) and the ($OH^-$) ions. When these ions are in equal proportions, the pH is a neutral 7. When there are more $H^+$ ions than $OH^-$ ions then the water is said to be "acid". And if the $OH^-$ ions are more than the $H^+$ ions, the water is said to be "alkaline." The pH scale goes from 0 to 14 and is logarithmic, which this means is that each step is ten times the previous. In other words, a pH of 4.5 is 10 times more acidic than pH of 5.5, 100 times more acidic than pH of 6.5 and 1,000 times more acidic than pH of 7.5.

We now can directly correlate between Voltage and pH as per the studies done by Nickola Telsa and Dr. Jerry Tennant. For example, the blood is strictly kept in the pH range of 7.35 ~ 7.45 and this is the same as saying a voltage of (–) 20 to (–) 25 mV.

The movement of electrons denotes an electrical charge. In your home, you have copper wires which act as conductors to carry this flow of electrons. If you switch on the circuit, the electrons move which then reflects as power, energy, and voltage – there is a donation of electrons, and the lights gets turned on. If the switch to that circuit is off, there are no electrons moving – no power or voltage.

Cells are designed to run at a voltage of (–) 20 to (–) 25 mV (Operating Voltage). This is the same as saying that cells must run in an environment of a pH of 7.35 to 7.45 [different sources vary slightly, so do not get lost about whether it is (–) 17 or (–) 20 mV and whether a pH of zero is (+) 400 or (+) 420 mV].

As said earlier, pH is also a measure of voltage. A pH of 0 is the same as (+) 400 mV. A pH of 14 is the same as (–) 400 mV. Cells normally operate at about pH of 7.2 or (–) 22 mV.



| pH | 0 | 7 | 14 |
|---|---|---|---|
| Voltage | +400 | 0 mV | -400 mV |

(Illustration is courtesy of
Dr. Jerry Tennant)

In the mortal body it is a different terrain, one that is always wettish – in solution; that solution can be an electron donor (alkaline pH) or an electron stealer (acidic pH). While these terms like electron donor and electron stealer may not be familiar to most people, once a voltage is measured using a sophisticated device it can be easily converted to a logarithmic scale called pH. This scale of measurement most people are very aware of. So, we now know that these terms can be used interchangeably.

Habitual health complaint and pain are nearly always associated with an acidic pH which is the same as saying that habitual health complaint and pain are nearly always associated with a loss of voltage. Health is associated with the presence of voltage which is the same as saying that healthy people have an alkaline pH.

In the body, being able to hold a charge of voltage is associated with minerals in general and particularly, calcium. This helps in cases of serious illness since alkaline pH does not favor growth of microorganisms. Cancer cells have trouble growing with alkaline pH as well.

The human cells of a normal body contain a lot of molecular oxygen and a slightly alkaline pH. The cancer cell has an acid pH and lack of oxygen.

If the environment is oxygen rich, Cancer cells cannot survive. If the pH rises slightly above 7.4 (salivary pH 6.7), the Cancer cells become dormant. At pH 8.5 (salivary pH 7.8) Cancer cells will die while the healthy cells will start living. Higher the pH reading of the fluid translates to more alkaline and oxygen rich environment.



Thus, it is mostly advantageous to push the pH above 6.5 if you are trying to overcome a chronic illness.

There is a special meter which can measure the voltage of a liquid. Known as the pH meter, it is used to know if the liquid is an electron donor or an electron stealer. The software of the meter converts the reading to a logarithmic scale called pH. The scale ranges from zero to 14. A pH of zero is a synonym of (+) 400 mV of electron stealer and (–) 400 mV of electron donor is a synonym of a pH of 14.

What Happens When Voltage Drops? Well, several bad things that happen as voltage begins to drop.

- Voltage drops: Fatigue; at (–) 15 mV, you are tired.
- Voltage Drops further: Oxygenation drops; as voltage drops more, several bad things get worse, ending with Cancer.

The voltage in water dictates the amount of oxygen that will dissolve in the water. Human cells consist of 70% water. So, when the voltage drops in our cells, they become oxygen deficient.

As oxygen levels drop, several other bad things happen – one of them being pain which is a symptom of low voltage. As voltage drops, we have chronic pain due to lack of oxygen.

The voltage necessary for the cells to work is provided by a rechargeable battery system which is housed inside our cells. When they are charged, they are called "ATP". When discharged they are called ADP (Adenosine di-phosphate). The battery system needs a battery charger which is the "Krebs cycle" or the "Citric Acid cycle." It prefers to run on fatty acids.

For every unit of fatty acid which passes through the Krebs cycle – if oxygen is present – you get enough electrons to charge up 38 of these ADP batteries. But if oxygen is low, for every unit of fatty acids processed by the Krebs cycle, you get enough electrons to charge up two of these ADP batteries. In such a scenario, our organs will become inefficient and will require much more fuel (fatty acids) to function. It is like a car going from 15 km/liter to 2 km/liter.

### Voltage Drop → Release of Pathogenic Digestive Enzymes

Another bad thing that happens has to do with infections. Each of us contains about a trillion "bugs". These bugs are suppressed if oxygen is present. However, as voltage and oxygen drop, the bugs wake up. They start releasing digestive enzymes which get dissolved in our cells to attack the nutrients. This starts the disease process.

These digestive enzymes get into your bloodstream and go throughout your body, causing damage at distant places. The enzymes travel throughout your system causing fever, nausea, muscle pain, headache and other symptoms and you might end up with strep throat.

They can scar anywhere else from your heart valves, knees, and other parts of your body.



The bacteria lose their cell membranes as voltage and oxygen drop further. This was described long back, in 1800's, by Antoine Bechamp as the cell-wall-deficient organisms. They have been noted by others (Enderlein, Naessens, Rife, Livingston, etc.) about every fifty years and given different names. The currently used name "L-forms," used by most microbiologists was termed by Lister Institute in Paris.

Because of the lack of cell membranes, the immune system cannot see them. Additionally, these do not cause the usual signs of infection like fever, higher white blood count and other markers.

These cannot be cultured either unless antibiotics are added to the culture media. Thus, it evades the consideration of the physicians that the infection has started the damage process. Moreover, antibiotics make them thrive. The only way to kill them is by raising the oxygen levels or using oxidative therapy (ozone, hydrogen peroxide, chlorine dioxide) or with frequencies.

*"It is my opinion that there is no such thing as an autoimmune disease. Such problems are really just the damage done by these cell-wall-deficient organisms, hiding somewhere in the body and doing damage at distant locations as well as locally. They will be hiding where the voltage is low. When you solve this problem, you will usually see the blood tests for autoimmune diseases go back to normal."*

*- Dr. Jerry Tennant*

So, when there is a drop in voltage to +30mV, cell-wall-deficient fungus shows up. They are always present when cancer occurs. In a specific acupuncture meridian, the polarity changes from electron donor to electron stealer.

Whenever voltage drops, the following steps always occur:

*Organ malfunction - chronic pain - lowered oxygen - lowered ATP (intercellular voltage) - infection with cell-wall-deficient organisms - fungus - cancer.*

The whole pathway is dependent upon lack of voltage.

## A Better Paradigm

Replacement of our cells that are constantly wearing out must be replaced. In every two days new cells are formed in the macula of our eyes.

The lining of our gut is replaced every three days. Replacement of the skin takes place in every six weeks and in every eight weeks, the liver is replaced.

It is when we lose this ability to make new cells that work that chronic disease occurs. Therefore, we must find out what does it take to make new cells that work.

Although cells run at (-) 25 mV, it takes (-) 50 mV to make a new cell. Chronic disease in almost all the cases is the lack of voltage necessary to make new cells. This along with the materials required to make new cells are also required and simultaneously addressing the toxins that damage the cells at the earliest.

So, the voltage in my thumb is (-) 25 mV. Now I hit it with a hammer and destroy some cells. My thumb will automatically go to (-) 50 mV.

When tissue is at (-) 50 mV, it dilates the arterial capillaries. The signs of inflammation are swelling, redness, pulsing pain, warmth etc.; and these are due to the dilated capillaries which is necessary for the body to provide the materials necessary to make the new cells.

We get busy and make new cells to replace those smashed by the hammer. Then the thumb goes back to (-) 25 mV and we are happy.

However, there is another possibility; we will be struck in the chronic disease state if we do not have the (-) 50 mV necessary to make new cells. The thumb does not have the voltage to work correctly, it is cold, pale, and has chronic pain. No matter how many pills we take or how much surgery we do, we cannot get well because we do not have the voltage necessary to make new cells.

If there is abnormal voltage, you will have pain. You will get a pulsating pain if the voltage is high. It hurts all the time when the voltage is low. The voltage can be corrected by using phosphoric acid (found in Coke) to lower the high voltage or using baking soda to raise the voltage. The pain will go away but it will come back because you have not corrected the reason the voltage was abnormal in the first place. In chronic disease, you must figure out why the battery pack to that organ or tissue cannot hold a charge.

## How Do Cells Normally Get Voltage?

So now we know the importance of maintaining a healthy (-) 25 mV cellular environments, the obvious question is "how do we actually influence the voltage of our cells?" It is to be ensured that our cells are optimally charged. We need to apply certain diet changes and lifestyle influences so that the new cells are optimally primed.

The following is a snapshot of these influential factors:

- Make sure that all nutrients necessary for making new cells that work are present.

- Remove all toxins and chemicals from your diet and lifestyle that inhibit this process. This means eating organic and non-GMO foods – only unprocessed food with a predominance of vegetable matter (raw foods are even better) ups your voltage.
- Not using any topical chemical based Personal Care and Home Care products.
- The 21$^{st}$ Century and its toxic environment is a big challenge here. The flow of voltage (electrons) is always from a higher voltage area to a lower voltage area. Just walking or standing barefooted on sand, grass or soil will help us to gather up voltage from the earth which is a big electromagnet.
- Swimming in a moving stream will increase your voltage.
- When two living things touch electrons flow from high to low. Contacting your healthy pet or a healthy tree will enable the movement of voltage into your energy system.
- Importantly, when you exercise, your muscles create electrons through what is called the piezoelectric effect. The muscles are rechargeable batteries and exercise is a major way to acquire electrons. These electrons are then transported to your organs and cells via 3 main pathways. The first is "Perineural Nervous System." Then the second is by way of "The Acupuncture Meridian System." The third is via the blood where the electrons are ionically transferred.

## You are your best defense against pathogens and disease!

The best way to optimize our chances of staying healthy is to raise our as narrated above voltage. This can be easily done as we are electric beings living in an electric Universe. This will strengthen our immune system; help our wounds to heal faster. Additionally, this will help boost our overall energy levels for optimal and sustained physical and mental activity.

## Drinking living water is one of the best ways to raise our voltage.

Living water is water that carries the full spectrum of life supporting enhancements. As in the molecular patterns of a solid quartz crystal, water also has a liquid crystalline phase; the water molecules create a repeating geometric structure. Although the molecules remain mobile, they appear to move together as a coherent whole. This live water forms an organized network that responds to its environment. Once the network has been established, it can carry signals and vibratory (frequency) information. This is like the way solid crystals are used in solid state technology.

Our bodies are 99% water by molecule and 70% water by volume. Please refer this link:

**https://www.prweb.com/releases/2014/03/ prweb11623245.htm**

So, it makes sense to ingest structured water having high negative ORP (Oxidation Reduction Potential) and infused with therapeutic levels of Molecular Hydrogen and using the above-mentioned techniques to raise our voltage.

# THE KEY TO GOOD HEALTH – HEXAGONAL WATER

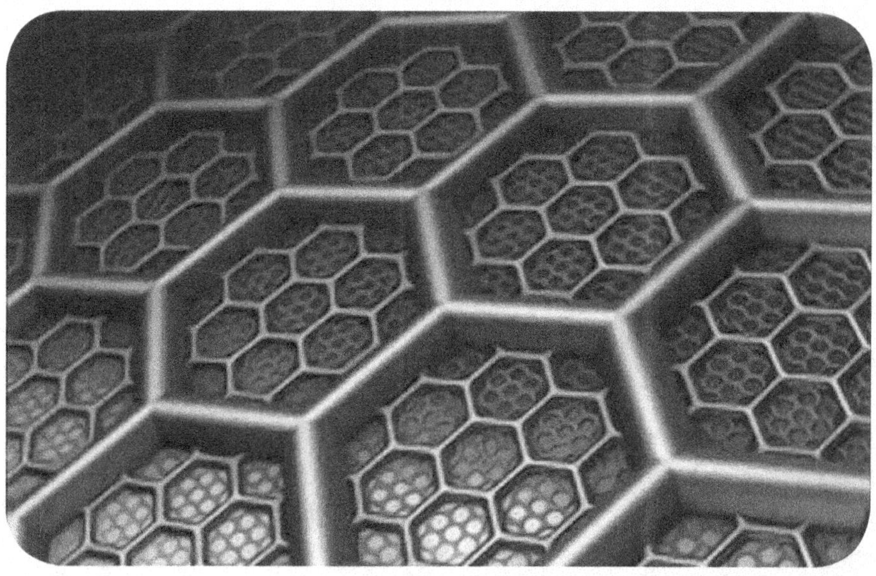

Hunza is a tribe that lives in Himalayan valley. These people have a life expectancy of around 120 years. Dr. Henri Conada, a Nobel Prize Winner, has extensively studied the Hunza water. He has spent decades there studying the water to determine what it was there in this water that played the most important role for their longevity. What he found was that the water had a different viscosity and surface tension.

Dr. Patrick Flanagan and others continued the research. Their findings showed that the water had a high alkaline pH, with a negative Redox Potential along with high colloidal mineral content.

Similar natural water properties and longevity are found in other remote unpolluted places such as the Shin-Chan areas of China, the

Caucasus in Azerbaijan, and in the Andes Mountains. In efforts to recreate the Hunza water, Japanese scientists investigated Russian electrolysis technology. To restructure the water electricity was used which gave the properties like that of Hunza water.

This functional water technology was first developed in Japan in the early 1950's and the experiments were first conducted on plants and animals. Several agricultural universities started full scale development of this technology. Research was also done on the effects of the acid water (from electrolysis) on plants. Japanese doctors started administering alkaline ionized water to their patients from the large sized ionizers installed in hospitals.

The Japanese Ministry of Health and Rehabilitation approved the water ionizers in January 1966 for medical therapeutics. Government of South Korea also approved them later as medical devices.

One of the world's leading authorities on the structure of water is Dr. Mu Shik Jhon (1932-2004). His book, "The Water Puzzle and the Hexagonal Key," summarizes years of research on the qualities and structure of water. Dr. John had an endless fascination with the characteristics of water, and ultimately on its effect on our health.

"The Water Puzzle and the Hexagonal Key" is not just someone else's ideas about water – collected over a period of 40 years and in simple terms it is a scientific documentation. There are people in some special areas that are known to live exceptionally long. The existence of a specific water structure, known as the "Hexagonal Water," is stated in this book. The book goes on to explain why this specific water structure is so energetically powerful; why it can move more efficiently within the body.

In 1986, Dr. John presented the "Molecular Water Environment Theory " at a symposium on cancer. As per this theory, if we replenish this structured water in our bodies, we will be increasing our vitality, slow down the aging process and prevent disease process. Aging is the result of the loss of Hexagonal Water from organs, tissues, and cells; an overall decrease in total body water, as per Dr. Jhon. The book shows us the science and the studies to back up these statements and he does it in a way that we can all understand. Dr. John's work has been the basis for technology that now produces Hexagonal Water, making it available for regular consumption.

For those of you who have been following the water revolution, with books like "You're Not Sick, You're Thirsty! "– Dr. F. Batmanghelidj (MD), and "The Message from Water" – Dr. Masaru Emoto, you will want "The Water Puzzle and the Hexagonal Key" to be your next book. This book has now been translated in 5 languages and has the power to revolutionize your thinking about water.

As per research, aging is associated with the loss of Hexagonal Water from organs, tissues and cells and an overall decrease in total body water. It is therefore suggested to start consuming Hexagonal Water to slow down the process of aging.

"Healing Springs" is the name given to those places all over the world that contain water with a high number of hexagonal structures. One such place is Lourdes in France. The inhabitants of these places are also known to live long disease-free lives. Ordinary tap water is seen to have large unorganized molecule size, which is not supportive of biological functions that take place in the human body. Since the hexagonal water has molecules which are smaller in size, it helps the biological functions to take place better.

Alkaline ionized water is hexagonal (structured). The easiest and most practical way to make this water at home is by Water Ionization. To lead a long and a life that is free of disease, we need to drink this hexagonal water in sufficient quantities daily.

# THE SECRET OF LONGEVITY OF "THE HUNZA TRIBE"

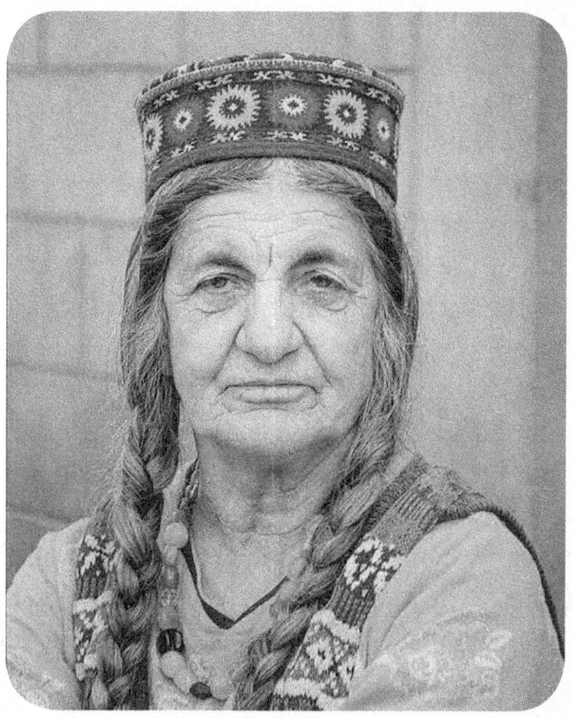

The Hunza People of Northern Pakistan are the longest living people on this planet. They are uniquely healthy and free of disease, and it is believed that their simple diet is the contributing factor to their longer lifespan. These include the organic food carefully grown and from the local glaciers which is their secret to health and long life.

Hunza drink water directly from glacial streams in the high Himalayas. The water is fresh, invigorating, life enhancing and free radical scavenging and is delicious. They drink alkaline and ionized water that naturally occurs. The longest lifespan of these people has been related to the water they drank and their natural diet.

Hunza people routinely live in the range of 120 to 140 years, in good health with virtually no cancer, degenerative disease, dental caries or bone decay. They remain robust, strong and are also able to bear children even in old age.

Research has proven conclusively that the major common denominator of the healthy long-living people is their local water.

These people are not the product of legend, nor are the countries they inhabit a mythical utopia. They call themselves the Hunzas and live in what has come to be known as the roof of the world – the mountain peaks of the Himalayas. The country with a population of just 30,000 is located at the extreme northern point of India.

Their water is life giving and provides health benefits that other types of drinking water cannot. Similar natural water properties and longevity are found in other remote unpolluted places such as the Kusatsu Onsen Hot Springs in Japan, the Lourdes Spring Water in France, in the Andes Mountains of Chile and many other places.

Maybe you are wondering: are the Hunzas really all that healthy? To find out these two cardiologists, Dr. Paul D. White and Dr. Edward G. Toomey made the difficult trip to the mountains of Hunza. They carried along with them a portable, battery-operated electrocardiograph.

They used the equipment to study 25 Hunza men, who were between 90 and 110 years old. Their blood pressure and cholesterol levels were also tested. As reported in the American Heart Journal for December 1964, none of the Hunzas showed any sign of high blood pressure, high cholesterol, or signs of coronary heart disease.

Dr. Allen E. Banik, an optometrist also wanted to see for himself whether the people there were as healthy as reported. He examined the eyes of some of Hunza's oldest citizens and found them to be perfect.

His report was published in Hunza Land (brought out by Whitehorn Publishing Co., in 1960).

The Hunzas have boundless energy and enthusiasm and are surprisingly serene. Their health is not characterized by the simple absence of disease, although that is quite an accomplishment. We can compare the average age of a westerner and that of a Hunza. A westerner who is considered extremely fit (though actually entering the zone of illness) would seem sickly, whereas a Hunza would be extremely fit.

The life expectancy of the average Westerner and that of the Indians is around 70 years. But for the Hunzas, it falls onto a different scale altogether. These people reach both their physical and intellectual maturity at the venerable age of one hundred which emphasizes the relative nature of what we refer to as normal.

No matter what the chronological age of the Hunzas is, they remain youthful in all ways. A Hunza is considered neither old nor even elderly even at one hundred years.

Is there a secret technique that allows these people to live so long and healthy? The answer is yes – the Hunzas do know something we do not. But there is not just one secret, there are many. And one among them is the water that they drink.

Holistic doctors and natural health practitioners are teaching us the fastest way to restore wellness is to quit putting into the body the things that have caused the physical problem to develop in the first place.

We have all now come to know that our bodies can heal themselves when given the right tools to do so. We all have been provided the most important immune system in our body. Most people do not understand how important the immune system is for our bodies to heal or how the immune system works.

The key to maintain good health is a strong immune system. Fresh air, pristine water, nutritious food, moderate exercise, sunshine, and optimum rest in the right balanced amounts are crucial.

There have been studies conducted on curative water sources such as Hunza water and glacial streams in the Himalayas and have discovered that these waters have been very alkaline and highly ionized.

The "fountain of youth" which people have been looking for has been literally found with ionized water. The earliest studies of water ionizer electrolysis dates to more than 60 years.

Our bodies are about 60-70 percent water. Research has shown with as little as a 1% loss of our body's water we experience loss of energy, metabolism, and ability to regulate body temperature. With as little as a 4% loss of the body's percentage of water, we get headaches and/or start to have more difficulty concentrating. And if the reduction falls below 10%, it is life-threatening.

Most people just attribute headaches, lack of energy and difficulty in concentrating to "aging". People do age, of course, but drinking enough water and the right water – the ionized water – can help determine how well you age.

There are growing numbers of people who are increasing their daily water intake and drinking ionized water which has resulted in feeling more energetic, staying alert and having better metabolism than before.

Ionized water in addition to providing the alkalinity buffers to the body, also provides an abundance of natural, simple, readily absorbable antioxidants to the body to help protect against the damaging effects of oxidation, which is the free-radical damage to the cells over the years. This helps hydration and in arresting the spiral of water-loss as we age.

Start feeling the difference right away by switching to Electrolyzed Reduced Water.

# DOES STOMACH ACID GET NEUTRALIZED WITH IONIZED ALKALINE WATER?

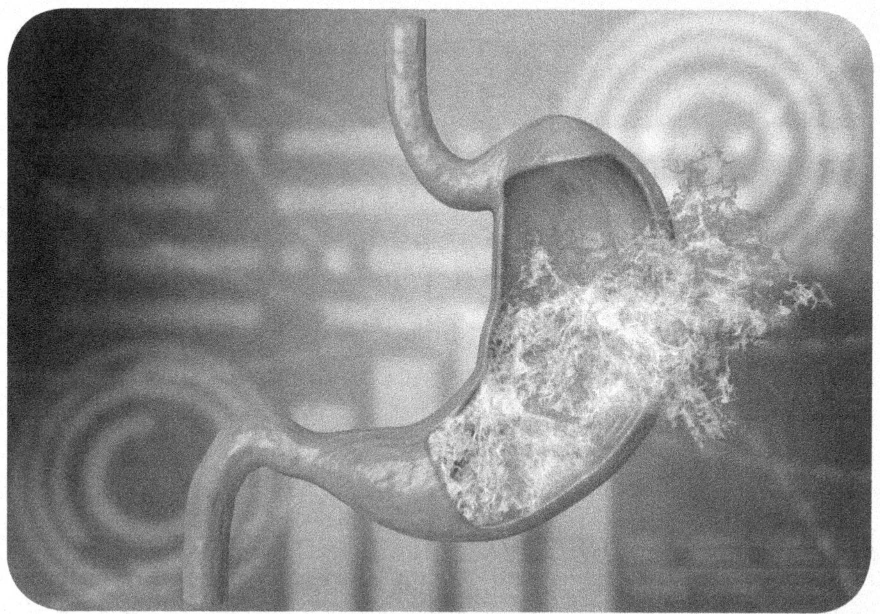

This is one of the questions most raised against alkaline water. Then why take the prescribed prescriptions if the stomach acid is so powerful? It can destroy the benefits of any medication.

Our body knows what is good for it. Stomach acid will try to destroy anything that is unhealthy for our body. To promote optimum health, nutrients, water, antioxidants, enzymes etc. are absorbed into our bodies.

Water on reaching our stomach does not become an acid. It, however, assists our bodies in clearing it of acids, so our body does not become acidic but remains alkaline (7.365 or better). The natural mechanism of our body helps our body to keep itself alkaline. The problem arises when we start putting wrong things inside us. Water is the most natural detoxification supplement available. As an example, we consume bottled water which is full of chemicals and plastics (a known fact). These are devoid of hydrating attributes. Tap water is neutral, bottled water sometimes is more acidic.

The natural waters of the world, from natural sources have a high pH level between 9.0 and 10.5 (making them alkaline). The purest water untouched by pollution, chemicals and waste is alkaline, which is why these are the best water to drink, by far.

## What happens to the water in the stomach if it does not become more acidic?

The inside of our stomach is acidic to digest food and kill the kinds of bacteria and viruses that come with food. The stomach pH value is maintained at around 4. The pH value inside the stomach goes up when we eat food and drink water, especially alkaline water.

There is a feedback mechanism in our stomach to detect when this happens. It commands the stomach wall to secrete more hydrochloric acid to bring the pH value back to 4. So, the stomach becomes acidic again. This means if we drink more alkaline water, more hydrochloric acid will be secreted to maintain the stomach pH value. It is like losing a battle.

However, when you understand how the stomach wall makes hydrochloric acid, your concerns will disappear. There is no hydrochloric acid pouch in our body. If there were, it would burn a hole in our body. The production of hydrochloric acid is done on an instantly-as-needed basis.

The ingredients in the stomach cell that make hydrochloric acid (HCl) are carbon dioxide ($CO_2$), water ($H_2O$), and sodium chloride (NaCl) or potassium chloride (KCl).

$$NaCl + H_2O + CO_2 = HCl + NaHCO_3, \text{ or}$$

$$KCl + H_2O + CO_2 = HCl + KHCO_3$$

Note that the byproduct of making hydrochloric acid is sodium bicarbonate ($NaHCO_3$) or potassium bicarbonate ($KHCO_3$), which goes into the bloodstream. Neutralization of the excess acids in the blood is done by these bicarbonates (the alkaline buffers). They dissolve solid acid wastes into liquid form. As they neutralize the solid acidic wastes, extra carbon dioxide is released, which is discharged through the lungs. These alkaline buffers get low as body ages, and this phenomenon is called acidosis. This is a natural occurrence as our body accumulates more acidic waste products.

By looking at the pH value of the stomach alone, it seems that alkaline water never reaches the body. But when you look at the whole body, there is a net gain of alkalinity as we drink alkaline water. Our body cells are slightly alkaline. To produce acid, they must also produce alkalinity and vice versa. It is just similar as a water ionizer which cannot produce alkaline water without producing acid water.

When the stomach pH value gets higher than 4, the stomach knows what to do to lower it. However, if the pH value goes below 4, for any reason, the stomach does not know what to do. That is why we take Alka-Seltzer (an antacid that gently breaks up and dissolves away the full feeling of acid indigestion and pain fast). It is alkaline and helps relieve acidic stomach gas pain. In this case, hydrochloric acid is not produced by the stomach wall and therefore, no alkaline buffer is being added to the blood stream.

Here is another example of a body organ that produces acid to produce alkalinity. After the food in the stomach is digested, it must come out to the small intestine. The food at this point is so acidic that it will damage the intestine wall. To avoid this problem, the pancreas makes alkaline juice (known as pancreatic juice). This juice is sodium bicarbonate and is mixed with the acidic food coming out of the stomach. From the above formulae, to produce bicarbonates, the pancreas must make hydrochloric acid, which goes into our bloodstream.

We experience sleepiness after a big meal (not during the meal or while the food is being digested in the stomach), when the digested food is coming out of the stomach; that is the time when hydrochloric acid goes into our blood. Hydrochloric acid is the main ingredient in antihistamines that causes drowsiness.

Alkaline or acid produced by the body must have an equal and opposite acid or alkaline produced by the body; therefore, there is no net gain. However, alkaline supplied from outside the body, like drinking alkaline water, results in a net gain of alkalinity in our body.

The above information shared is not designed to diagnose, treat, or to be used in lieu of qualified medical attention. These little pearls of wisdom come from actual application of the various types of electrolyzed reduced water by me personally for more than 6 years of continuous use and innumerable personal testimonies from patients under supervision of his/her personal physician, based with a specific outcome that is expected and monitored.

(Note: This chapter has been compiled from various sources available on the internet)

# PROFESSIONAL ATHLETES AND HYDROGEN WATER

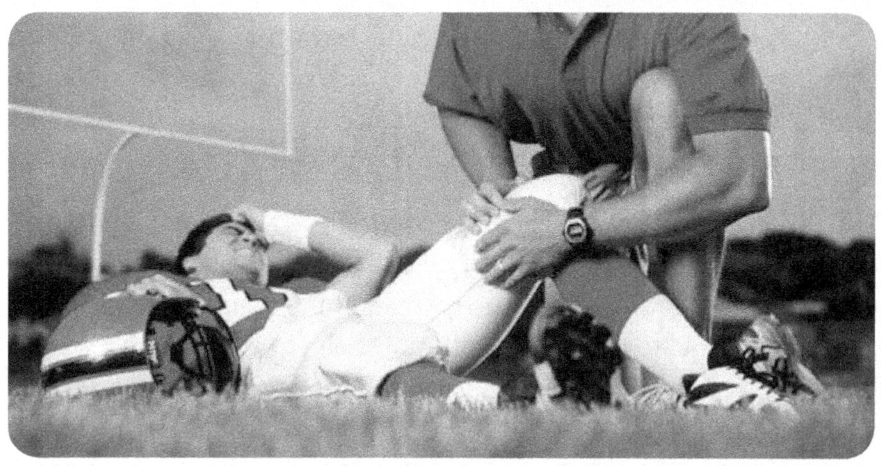

[Image Credit: Copyright: (c) Tony Garcia]

The purpose of this chapter is to lay out an invitation from a global community of highly respected doctors, scientists, and medical researchers to transform the world of high-contact sport into a much safer workplace for all athletes to perform. Therefore, we stand ready to educate and help integrate Hydrogen Water Therapy into any level of size of sports league and/or organizations for the benefit of all parties.

One of the greatest worries for all professional athletes is a major injury to their spine, limb bone, joint, knee, hip, or shoulder. Fortunately, Hydrogen water can potentially rescue our dedicated athletes from such career-ending injuries.

There are also 7 other areas of concern for professional athletes:

- Maximum oxygen uptake
- Reliable, consistent energy levels
- Muscle fatigue
- Lactic acid build-up
- Faster post-workout or post-game recoveries
- Inflammation
- Micro injuries to bones, joints, muscles, connective tissues, and nerve, including brain tissues and nerves.

We have access to many scientific studies on the above seven areas of concern. One human study[3] of elite male soccer players have been published in 2012. This real, in-the-field human study concluded, in part, that adequate hydrogen hydration helped reduce "pre-exercise blood lactate levels" and improved "exercise-induced decline of muscle fatigue."

It is no longer a theory that hydrogen water therapy can in most cases prevent or treat all the above seven areas professional athletes constantly worry about. Just imagine, as a professional athlete knowing having perhaps, the ultimate edge in your category of sports. Imagine waking up every day with confidence knowing your hydration protocol is back by over 1,000 scientific studies proving Hydrogen water is protecting, repairing and delivering therapeutic properties to your entire body at a Nano level.

Every month, more professional athletes are adding Hydrogen Water to their hydration program. Some of the biggest names in professional sports already have one hydrogen edge. However, without proper education and training by a "Molecular Hydrogen Advisor" and "Nano Hydrogen Specialist" … most athletes may experience no more than 50% of its benefits.

---

[3]  **https://www.ncbi.nlm.nih.gov/pubmed/22520831**

## Sports and energy drinks, and other Supplements – the short-term fix to a bigger problem!

We give in to the marketing campaigns and convenience in exchange for drinks that can seriously harm our body's long-term health. Let us group these together with just some of their dangers:

- Stimulants like Caffeine
- Sugar, high levels, from GMO corn, high fructose corn syrup
- Excessive B Vitamins
- Artificial Sweeteners (Aspartame, Sucralose and Saccharin)
- Phenylalanine (can behave as a neurotoxin) – ADD/ADHD
- Citric acid (Preservative)
- Potassium Sorbate (Preservative)
- Sodium Benzoate, Benzoic Acid and Benzoate (Preservative)
- Colorings (chemical dyes such as Sunset Yellow)

Hundreds of studies link excessive stimulants and sugar to heart problems and diabetes. Two studies showed Potassium Sorbate (PS) can mess with DNA. One more study proved PS is toxic to human blood cells. Another study revealed PS mixed with ascorbic acid (Vitamin C) caused mutagenicity and DNA damaging activity.

When Benzoic Acid (BA) is combined with Nitric Acid, the highly carcinogenic benzene is produced. Few helpful resource links are embedded in the following,[4] to help us move away from their dangers.

A new category of supplements has now recently emerged and are literally flooded in the supermarkets. These are the Portable Mixes and Electrolytes and are termed as "Water Enhancers" to catch the attention of the most venerable section of the consumers, the younger generation. These are designed to add flavor, sweetness and, in some

---

4 https://www.thehealthyhomeeconomist.com/sports-drinks-hide-aspartame/

products, a few healthy minerals. Some are powders and others are package as liquids then squeeze bags of plastic containers.

If suppose one major brand named "SuperWater" sells their flavored enhancer drops. Notice what are the ingredients included in it. Probably, it will contain:

- Citric Acid
- Sucralose
- Potassium Sorbate
- Red 40 and Yellow 6

What is the goal of "SuperWater" – from a well-known branded company? Their advertisements say, "add our drops to your clean pure bottled water." Their marketing is crafted to get us buy a new product and buy more of their bottled water to increase the sales and profits. The potential dangers of these ingredients, when combined with each other, have been narrated earlier.

> *"Parents who give children energy drinks might well be giving them cocaine."*
>
> *- James Oliver (Celebrity Chef and Author)*

Many dieticians and naturopathic doctors warn against using these water enhancers and energy drinks.

> *"Don't fall the healthy hype… many of these drink mixes are loaded with fake, chemical additives."*
>
> *- Johannah Sakimura, RD[7]*

---

[5] **https://www.everydayhealth.com/columns/johannah-sakimura-nutrition-sleuth/water-enhancers-dont-live-up-to-name**

## Cocktail of Death: The Top Ingredients in Energy Drinks

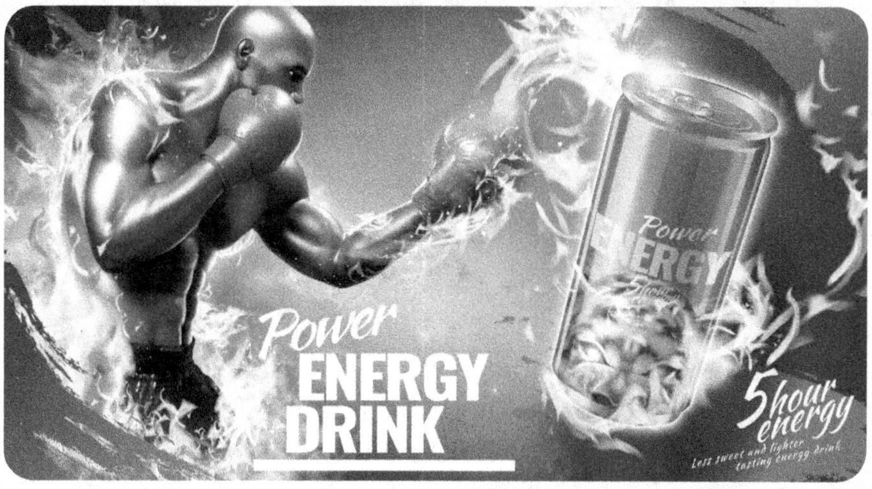


Are energy drinks killing us softly? Many studies have linked energy drinks with Heart Arrhythmia, Irregular Heart Palpitations, Increased Blood Pressure, Dehydration, Gastrointestinal Problems, Chest Pain, Dizziness, Headache and even Death.[6]

What about all the electrolyte products we can now add to our water? The ones available in the market and certified by authorities are the cause of health issues narrated above as they are devoid of the trace minerals required for rehydration and absorption.

Regardless of your present health status or age, it is always advisable to stay away from the so-called energy drinks. If you have a history of high blood pressure, heart problems, or if you are pregnant, it is always better to avoid these – even coffee, caffeine tea and alcohol for that matter. There is no place for energy drinks in the diet of a child or adolescent.

---

[6] https://www.seattleorganicrestaurants.com/vegan-whole-food/toxic-ingredients-in-energy-drinks.php

The above quote says it all.

Professional athletes, especially those are associated with high-contact professional sports, are invited to embrace this Global movement towards injury prevention / quick recovery with the "Hydrogen Water Therapy." The research and scientific evidence are both irrefutable and undeniable. A massive body of studies that span over 40 years indicates that this revolutionary therapy with virtually universal application for all professional sports is available today.

Let this therapy be included as the primary adjunct to the existing injury and concussion protocols... at all levels of high-contact sports, including public and private school programs. There is virtually little to no risk to begin adding Hydrogen Therapy, even on a trial basis, to the existing injuries and concussion protocols. The reward is essentially unlimited potential preventive and therapeutic benefit for all athletes.

Visit: **www.molecularhydrogeninstitute.com/studies**

# HELPFUL TIPS FOR DRINKING MOLECULAR HYDROGEN

Here are a few tips that may help improve or even maximize your personal "Hydrogen Water Therapy." The goal is to simplify drinking and eating so we can enjoy both with ease.

## The "20-Minute 1-2-3 Method/ Guideline" for drinking Hydrogen Water

On waking up, drink 2 glasses of freshly Ionized Hydrogen Water on an empty stomach. It is advised to wait for at least 20 minutes each time we drink 1 or 2 glasses of Alkaline Water before consuming food. We must allow our pH sensitive pyloric valve to open wide and let this very safe medical grade water to quickly flow through our valve into our upper GI tract.

After 20 minutes of first drinking our two glasses on empty stomach, we should aim to drink the second round of 2 glasses of fresh Hydrogen water. This gives us our daily "foundation" of hydrogen gas and micro-minerals that is alive in the alkaline water with millions of antioxidants.

Why is the 20-minute wait guideline so important? It is advised not to consume too much water and food together. There is a well-designed "sensor" mechanism with intelligent feedback loops in our stomach and the pyloric valve. When our stomach senses any food, it immediately interprets that food as a meal and produces acids to digest our "meal" … even if it is only a snack.

Very important: Drinking high-alkaline water with a meal or too soon after a meal can have a negative impact on our stomach's ability to efficiently digest food. Remember… we need our stomach to be acidic for healthy digestion. If at all required to drink water with the meals, just drink a bit little of the 7.0 neutral pH water (free of hundreds of contaminants) from the water ionizer.

How long do you wait after a snack or meal? It is vital to allow our stomach enough time to digest food using its well-designed digestive system. Our stomach must remain acidic for healthy digestion. Digestion gets hindered by drinking lots of water with any meal. If we must drink to swallow a pill or a portion of our food, just drink a little (sip) of the pH neutral "purified" water.

The following is the 20-minute / 1-2-3 Method:

- After a **light snack or meal**: wait for 1 hour for your stomach to digest food. After this, drink one or two glasses of Hydrogen water.
- After an **average size meal**: wait for 2 hours for your stomach to digest food. After this, drink one or two glasses of Hydrogen water.
- After a **heavy meal** (especially with hard-to-digest proteins is like red meat), wait for 3 hours. Then resume Hydrogen hydration.

## Before Meals:

Drinking Hydrogen water 20 minutes before every meal can help us distinguish between thirst and hunger. Many people do not chew while eat as much. Consumption of Hydrogen Water 20 minutes the meal helps us to chew more completely rather simply gulp down the food. It is also a good idea to drink 1 to 2 glasses of Hydrogen water 2-3 hours after each meal. In this way, Hydrogen water is being consumed throughout the day.

## Taking Medications:

Medication should be taken with the non-ionized water with pH 7.0. Hydrogen may have a more potent effect. It has been recommended that medication be taken at least 30 minutes before or after drinking Hydrogen water. You should work with your doctor or health practitioner when drinking Hydrogen water. Some people have reduced or eliminated certain medications under a doctor's care, supervision, and approval.

## Taking Nutritional Supplements:

Hydrogen water is perfect for taking quality nutritional supplements. Hydrogen aids in a more complete assimilation (absorption) of their nutrients.

## Taking Acidic Beverages, including Tea and Coffee:

Brewing coffee, tea or making other acidic beverages with the high alkaline (pH 9-10) Hydrogen water can reduce acidity, improve taste, and provide some hydrogen benefits. Making ice cubes with higher alkaline (pH 9-10) hydrogen water can give some benefits as described above. Avoid plastic trays and only use food grade stainless steel ice trays.

## Method of Drinking:

- Sit down and drink water always. Avoid drinking standing.
- Avoid gulping all the water at once.
- Drink room temperature water, warm is even better.
- Drink water first thing in the morning.

# CHLORINE IN YOUR WATER – WHY YOU SHOULD BE WORRIED?

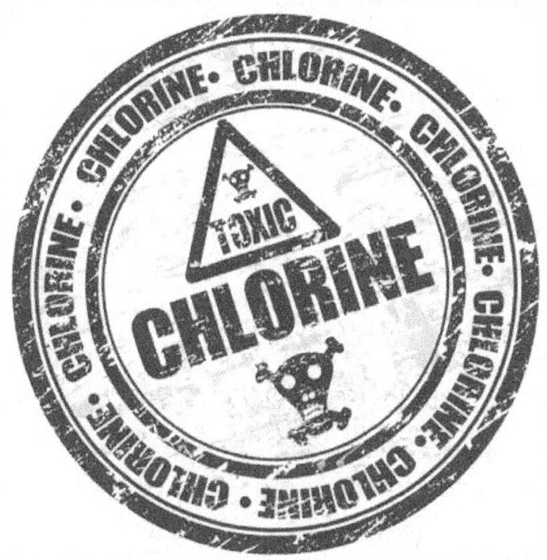


Chlorine is highly detrimental to human health and this chapter will highlight the dangers of bathing in Chlorinated water.

We are getting our daily doses of Chlorine with our waters without even knowing and it is creating havoc on our bodies, our immune and endocrine system, and others.

Halogens are a family of non-metal elements on the periodic table that share similar chemical properties. Three of these halogens are toxic to our bodies. These three toxic elements include Fluorine (think Fluoride), Chlorine, and Bromine. Another halogen is Iodine, which is the only halogen that the human body needs.

Iodine – the one "good" halogen is needed for the creation of thyroid hormones. Just like with thyroid hormone, every cell in your body also has an Iodine receptor. Iodine is a critical nutrient for thyroid health. Iodine helps prevent further cancer by improving immunity, and by helping to induce "apoptosis" (self-destruction) of cancerous cells, while not destroying your healthy cells.

The other three Halogens – Fluoride, Chlorine and Bromine are toxic in them, but are also highly detrimental because our body's Iodine receptors might get blocked thus preventing our body from absorbing the Iodine it needs.

Chlorine is the most common halogen added in our Municipality Water to reduce pathogenic bacteria and is to be avoided at all costs. Of course, the quality of your drinking water is a major factor in your health and well-being.

Chlorine is everywhere. It is in tap water, bath shower, swimming pools, gyms, hot tubs, and foods – both cooked and raw, cleaned with supply water. If you soak in a hot bath for 15 minutes you absorb chlorine as if you drink one whole full liter of the water. So, you can very well imagine if you in the pool for an hour.

We are aware that bathing is critical to health and that our skin is the primary connection to the world. It is the largest organ; it filters toxins; it has very high absorption rate; the sebaceous glands are susceptible to toxins; hair follicle can absorb toxins deep into your systems, blood vessels and lymph's.

This means the filtration of your shower and bath water may be even more important than the water you drink!

The free radicals in chlorinated water have been linked to liver malfunction and weakening of the immune system. There are lots of evidence to prove how Chlorine can make a damaging effect on the beneficial human gut bacteria.

Chlorine is a powerful antimicrobial agent and is an effective pesticide against many different strains of bacteria. The compounds in disinfected water may be able to reach your gut, not only through your drinking water, but also by being absorbed through your skin and inhaled whenever you take a bath or shower.

Chlorinated water for bathing and showering poses a major risk of cancer. Research supports this statement. This suggests that the health risks associated with Chlorine may be more related to absorption through the skin and through inhalation.

Inhalation of Chlorine vapors from a single 10-minute shower has been shown to be greater than the amount of Chlorine ingested from the average two liters of water you may drink. The damage to the linings of the gut is evident.

Chlorine is an "Iodine Antagonist," which means our Thyroid glands are directly affected ultimately leading to shut down of our Endocrine System.

There is a study listed on PubMed titled: Human respiratory uptake of chloroform and haloketones during showering: **https://pubmed. ncbi.nlm.nih.gov/15138448/**

Chlorine reacts with other natural compounds to form the byproduct known as Trihalomethanes (THMs). These are highly carcinogenic and trigger cell damage. Women with breast cancer have up to 60% THMs in their fat tissues. Cancer risk among people using chlorinated water is as much as 95% higher than the water free of chlorine.

These disorders often have widespread symptoms, affect multiple parts of the body, and can range in severity from mild to very severe and include overproduction of growth hormone, hyperthyroidism, hypothyroidism, and others.

We take care of our drinking water by installing costly RO which removes Chlorine. But the RO water by itself is the cause of disease process as it makes the water acidic. But we bathe, generally wash our vegetables and fruits, and do all our daily activities with the supply water.

The fast absorption of chlorine in our body and the produce we wash with supply water can be shown as a live demonstration. It is strongly suggested seeing the live demo as to how we are getting our daily doses of Chlorine with our waters without even knowing which is creating havoc on our bodies, our immune and endocrine system, and others.

Bathing is critical to health and healing. We all know that our skin is the primary connection to the outside world.

Get introduced to a whole new World of "Onsen." Literally, Onsen means "hot spring." In fact, these are natural hot water baths rich in beneficial minerals. Just Google "Onsen" and you will be taken to a new world of healing.

In the earlier times, people had limited knowledge on health and medications. Hot springs were used as a sacred place where people could cure their diseases and injuries.

Onsen contains different minerals specified by the "Onsen Law of 1948" in Japan. The law states that the spring water must be 25 degrees centigrade or above and should contain certain levels of mineral content.

The Ministry of Health in Japan regulates these Medical Hot Springs. "Pharmacologically" by components of the minerals and salts; "Thermally" by the heat; "Buoyancy" by the weightless relaxation; "Hydrodynamic Pressure" increases the blood flow to the lymph's; "Changing Environment" gives the "Womb Effect."

Pharmacologically – (a) "Sulfur" helps conditions of dry skin, chronic dermatitis, eczema, psoriasis (b) "Copper" helps in anemia and menstrual conditions (c) "Radium" helps in joint and muscle pains, neuralgia (d) "Carbon Dioxide" helps in constipation and high blood pressure (e) "Sodium Bicarbonate and Chloride" helps in wound healing and gastrointestinal disorders (f) "Silica" helps maintain the skin soft.

Thermal mineral content under hydrodynamic water pressure increases blood flow to lymphatic and builds cardiovascular integrity. It helps in controlling thyroid, fibromyalgia, rash, eczema, psoriasis, acne, and hair loss.

Noboribetsu, is a city in the Northern Island of Hokkaido's which has the most famous hot spring resort, offering different kinds of thermal waters that are considered among Japan's best and most effective. These contain Tufa, a calcium mineral stone, which directly comes from the Futamata Radium Hot Spring in Hokkaido, Japan. These stones render the regular tap water into waters akin to the hot springs.

Please view a short video titled "Snow Monkeys soak in Hot springs" **https://www.youtube.com/watch?v=6FzrsIOnIpo**

A new exclusive Home Spa System from a Japanese company, which is an Original Equipment Manufacturer (OEM), transforms your ordinary bathroom into a natural hot spring resort.

Treat yourself to a soothing hot spring experience with this ultimate home spa system!

The system is easy to install and has (a) external filters – which remove Chlorine, trihalomethanes, phenols, sediments, odor, taste and organic wastes (b) contains Neodymium Magnets (which are rare earth magnets) – these are high intensity magnets that breaks water molecule to the small clusters and activates the water (c) contains Ceramic Internal Cartridge – that generates mildly alkaline water.

It can produce a continuous stream of healthy ionized mineral water. It removes almost 100% of chlorine and other harmful substances in your tap water, and adds safe, moisturizing minerals that are healthy for your skin and hair.

# SURVIVING IN UNCERTAIN TIMES

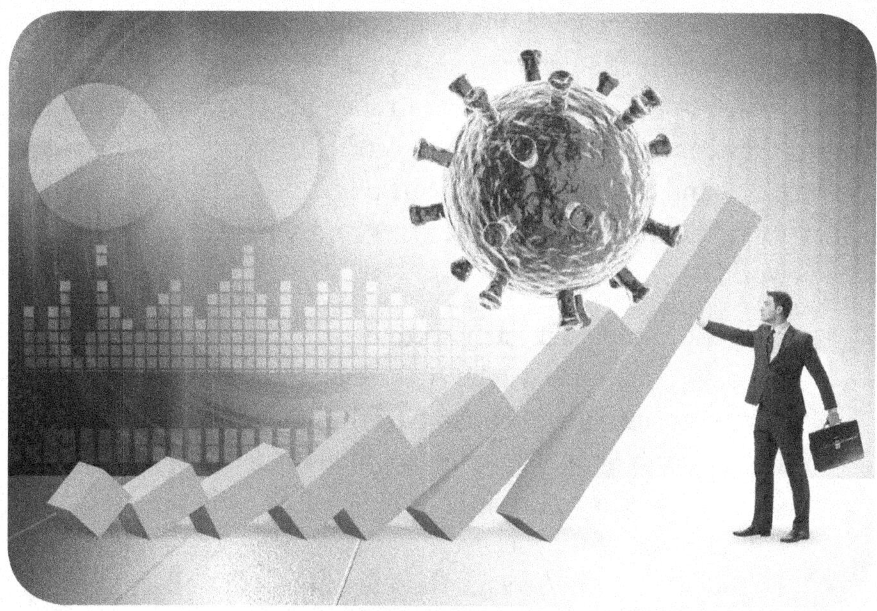

We are passing through very difficult times post pandemic situations and staring at a potential global recession. There is a total uncertainty globally. All these can lead to stress which may be at an all-time high. What can be the implications of this event which will affect your career, family, team members? What will be the financial situation, the economy and many more?

And when this stress leads to health problems which might eventually kill you, will you begin to search high and low for an explanation and solution to your dilemma. Until then, you just cannot appreciate the emotionally draining impact of a visit to the hospital, especially in this present scenario or for that matter a visit to your doctor's clinic will be on you and your entire family and the ultimate pronouncement of his or her serious findings. Let us hope you or anyone you care for never confronts such a situation – which thousands are now facing daily.

We spend enormous amounts on medical research and correctly so. However, if you look at any of the recent publications you will see page upon page of explanation about diseases that kill; Yet when the authors of these reach to the point of having to shed light on the cause of the disease, they confess – "etiology unknown."

Only Diet and Medicines will not help!!

Let us take a hard look at the facts and what we are facing in today's world:

- It is estimated that each second or third man in this new generation of today will be affected by Cancer in their lifetime. Fifty years ago, it was one in twenty-five.
- In 1900, only about 5% of the population died of Heart Disease, Cancer, or Diabetes. Today, 95% of us will die from any combination of these causes.
- In the last about 20 years, despite billions of dollars spent on research, Cancer has become the number 2 killer.
- Every year a few millions of women feel fine before being diagnosed with Breast Cancer who feels fine. A sizable number of these women eventually die.
- For majority of men and women with heart disease, a fatal attack is their first symptom.
- One in three people will get Diabetes in their lifetime – some starting as early as 12 years old or younger.
- One in fifty is stricken with Autism now. It was one in Ten Thousand 25 years ago.
- Dementia and Alzheimer are getting right up there with Diabetes and Cancer.

We become sick as our body's own defense system gets weakened. This is caused by the body becoming too acidic and overly inflamed. We are all dehydrated to an extent that feeds both acidity and inflammation.

Dr. Otto Warburg discovered the root cause of Cancer in 1923 for which he was awarded the Nobel Prize for his findings that Cancer needs an "Acidic and Inflamed" environment to thrive.

Acidity and Inflammation are the root cause of nearly every disease out there. Heart Disease is caused by Inflammation. Autoimmune Disease including Lyme, Lupus, MS and on and on, are all products of inflammation. Diabetes, Ketoacidosis, is an acidity issue that causes inflammation. This is the inflammation buildup caused by Diabetes.

Now let us look at what it takes to prevent these diseases and get our body back in balance.

First, we need to understand how we become Acidic and Inflamed. So let me address the acidity issue.

Think of your body as if it were your garden. Garden soil needs to have proper mineral and nutrient balance for our garden to thrive. The body is the same.

Our body is constantly feeding the blood with vital minerals which are Calcium, Magnesium and Potassium. The blood must maintain a level in alkalinity or pH of 7.365 more or less.

If we are not replacing the mineral the body uses, the body becomes more and more acidic. The important thing is that it must be in the right form for the body to use.

We need to stay away from eating or drinking overly acidic foods and drinks. A carbonated soft drink is only one point less acidic than battery acid. Why do we drink it? Sugar and artificial sweeteners are another killer. As our body becomes more acidic, the more our defense system gets weakened.

The inflammation part is a little more complicated. Inflammation is caused by Oxidative Stress.

Oxidative Stress is caused when oxidants in our body overpower the antioxidants in our body. We can easily see this by cutting an apple in half and setting it on the table for a couple hours. It turns brown, which is the process of oxidation.

So, we know oxidation comes from air. Foods are also oxidant. There are fruits and vegetables rich in antioxidants such as blueberries. Proteins are usually always oxidative. So again, this is a matter of balancing the right foods.

Bottled Waters are very oxidative. Tap waters are even more on account of chemical additives. Our tap waters are as oxidative as carbonated soft drinks due to the amount of chemicals used to treat our water supply. Chlorine is extremely oxidative. That is how it kills bacteria.

Since there are oxidants all around us, antioxidants in large amounts are needed to balance the oxidants. Considering how polluted our air and water supply has become, it may be impossible to eat enough antioxidant foods to offset the oxidants unless you move to the mountains somewhere where the air is pure, and the water is fresh, clean and pristine.

A simple change of your water can bring your life back to balance.

# HYDROGEN – ALTERNATIVE FUEL TO ALTERNATIVE MEDICINE!

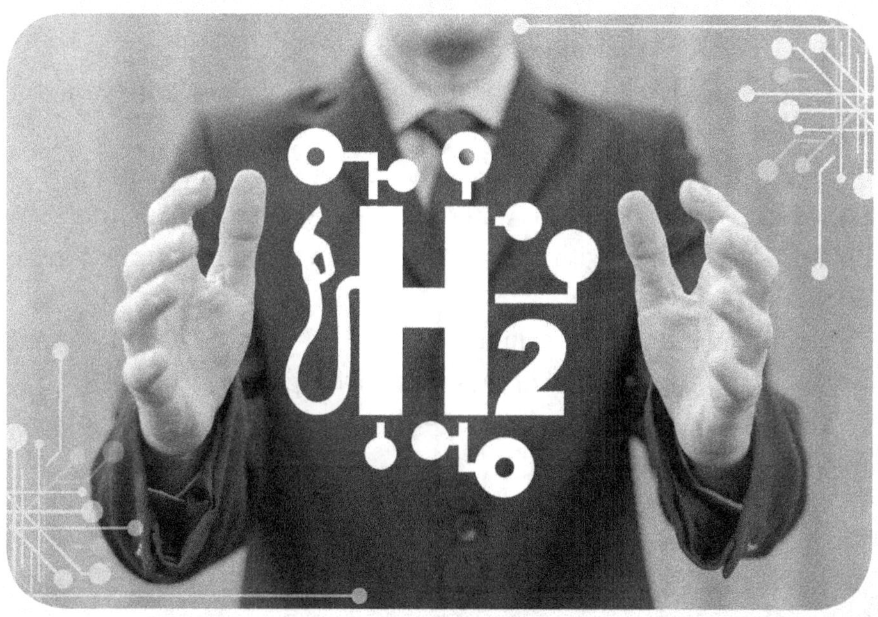

Hydrogen gas ($H_2$) has been extolled for its use in "green energy" as an alternative fuel, but biomedical research over the past decade suggests it also has therapeutic biological benefits. For example, the preliminary 1000+preclinical and clinical studies have reported hydrogen to have antioxidant, anti-inflammatory, anti-allergy, anti-obesity, and anti-aging effects.

http://www.molecularhydrogeninstitute.com/hydrogen-alternative-fuel-to-alternative-medicine?fbclid=IwAR3iJZrLaudzZNnWFGWJfVhvmdrXnLJURssZp1yLCTwulb20wbl69ycifnI

There are 321 studies on this amazing reactive oxygen species (ROS) scavenger: **https://www.ncbi.nlm.nih.gov/pmc/articles/PMC4610055/**

Portable Hydrogen Water Bottles is the latest thing being sold in the stores with prices starting from Rs. 2,000. Also, Hydrogen Infused Packed Drinking Water now available from Rs. 500 per liter.

There is absolutely no therapeutic value of $H_2$ at a low concentration which is what you get from all these above.

In scientific literature, to get the therapeutic value of $H_2$, the hydrogen gas dissolved in water should range from 0.5 mg/L to 1.6 mg/L, or more [with most studies using a concentration near 1.6 mg/L].

For explanation of the solubility of various gases in water followed by a focus on the solubility of molecular hydrogen, click:

**http://www.molecularhydrogeninstitute.com/concentration-and-solubility-of-h2**

Here is another quick way to test the presence of $H_2$… use a lighter. Hydrogen is the smallest element of the periodic table. In the gaseous state it is flammable and burns with a pop sound. When we say hydrogen is "burning", it is undergoing a chemical reaction where it combines with oxygen to form water releasing a lot of energy.

$$2H + O \rightarrow H_2O + energy$$

Lots of energy is released by hydrogen when it combusts, and most of this energy is released in the form of heat.

Heat causes gasses to expand, and since a lot of heat is released the gaseous mixture (hydrogen, oxygen remaining from, and water vapor liberated from the reaction) and the air adjacent to it expand very quickly, so quickly that the gas molecules break the sound barrier (with a pop sound).

You deserve the best, not some marketing gimmicks. Do not fall for those gimmicks! Make your own unlimited supply of real hydrogen water at home daily for pennies. With a onetime nominal investment on your health for the "Essential Kitchen Equipment," you are literally covered for all your hydration needs. Remember, your body will last much more than that fancy car.

The Electrolyzed Reduced Water (with other waters), from the "Water Ionizing Generator" which I have been using since the last 6 years has been approved as a Medical Device by the Japanese Ministry of Labor and Welfare. Additionally, these Ionizers have been given the Seal of Approval by "The Japanese Association of Preventive Medicine" for Adult Lifestyle Diseases. This association comprises of more than 6,500 Japanese Physicians and Surgeons. These are also GOLD SEAL Certified by the Water Quality Association (WQA), USA. Being an Original Equipment Manufacturer, they are associated right from the research, and finally till the distribution of their products to the end users globally. With a 48-year history, they initially provided ionized, alkalized water to hospitals in Japan since 1974 for 20 years before being introduced as a domestic unit.

The flagship model which I use generates a Molecular Hydrogen with a concentration of over 1.3 mg/L at the 9.5 pH setting (and this can be shown at a Live Demonstration using a Hydrogen Meter). The premium model gives a concentration of 1.6 mg/L. It is strongly suggested to drink the freshly made Hydrogen infused water with other unique properties straight from the ionizer, to get the maximum benefits.

## Afterword: Share the knowledge about Molecular Hydrogen

Hopefully, this book must have transformed your thoughts, beliefs and assumptions on this humble molecule called "Hydrogen." So, the question which now comes to our mind is – "why Molecular Hydrogen is not on top of the food chain especially when it can address to almost all health challenges?"

The reason is that even with its great potential medical applications, we are still in the early days of understanding other factors involved in the functionality of this molecule, especially as a bioactive molecule in humans. Although the research has seemingly proved promising in animal cells, more chemical and long-term trials are still in progress to fully confirm what we know about its efficiency in the human body.

Healthcare is always changing. Past changes have been driven by science, innovation, and technology. Today's changes are mainly economic; healthcare costs too much for too long. Healthcare providers of to discover how to deliver better care at a lower cost, or we will torpedo the economy and put our most vulnerable populations at risk.

I am fortunate on being a part of many great organizations during my journey of 18 years, initially as a wellness consultant and then eventually as an intellectual distributor and trainer in the Direct Selling Industry, both in India and Abroad. I am grateful to everyone whose life I have been able to touch, as in return, I have been enriched many folds.

We are always driven by our purpose to improve the quality of life for every person who comes through our doors and elevate the community we touch. There is no greater love than that of good health and your continued dedication to our very own people is very much recognized and appreciated. Through the lending of our expertise, our time or even just our kind smiles, we can turn a potentially traumatic experience of people into a warm memory.

I am very fortunate to serve all my clients with compassion. Please know that I am extending my sincerest gratitude to all of you, and I look forward to your continued success in the coming years. I can guide you with safer alternative alternate modes of treatments which can help resolve the health issues of you and your loved ones (if any), along with supplementing your current diet best suited to you.

The best is yet to come!

# ABOUT THE AUTHOR

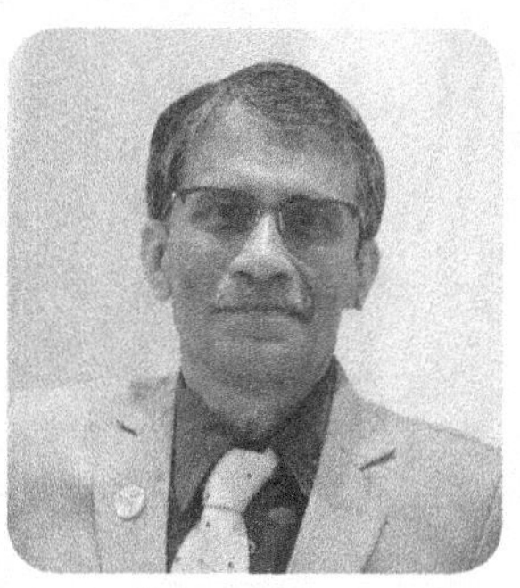

Dr. Debi Prasad Acharjya got his basic education from Christ Church Boy's School, Jabalpur (Madhya Pradesh) and graduated from St. Aloysius College (Jabalpur University, Madhya Pradesh) in B.Sc. by being a Gold Medalist. Later he completed his Post Graduate Diploma in Systems Management from NIIT, Kolkata. He is a Certified Law of Attraction Basic Practitioner from Global Sciences Foundation, USA. He is a certified Emotional Freedom Technique (EFT) Consultant from Vitality Living College, UK and also has a Certificate in Medical Transcription.

He is a Graduate of "Landmark Forum." Dr. Acharjya is a former officer of Canara Bank, one of the most respected financial institutions of India. He also has a Diploma in Cellular Nutrition Therapy (DCNT) from "The Open International University for Complementary Medicines", Colombo, Sri Lanka. For his significant contribution in the field of "Wellness and Well Being," he has been awarded Honorary Doctorate by the Medicina Alternativa, affiliated to The Open International University of Colombo, Sri Lanka.

He is an International Hydration Specialist and has been awarded the certificate of "Hydrogen Advisor" from the "Molecular Hydrogen Institute (MHI)." The institute is the epicenter of hydrogen education and training and is the leading educational source for individuals interested in accurately sharing the scientific evidence regarding the therapeutic benefits of $H_2$ gas.

As an Ambassador of Global Health and Wellness and with years of experience and the multitude of resources, he guides people to understand what exactly is needed to acquire a healthy life at any age! As a Wellness Coach he has transformed lives of thousands of people. Working with Dr. Acharjya is a learning experience; say his beneficiaries with a sense of pride and fulfillment.

**Web:** https://www.successlifecreation.com